It Really
Does Happen
To a Vet

JOE INGLIS

It Really Does Happen To a Vet

SIDGWICK & JACKSON

To my long-suffering wife Emma for everything.

First published 1999 by Sidgwick & Jackson
an imprint of Macmillan Publishers Ltd
25 Eccleston Place, London SW1W 9NF
Basingstoke and Oxford
www.macmillan.co.uk

Associated companies throughout the world

ISBN 0 283 06343 2

1 3 5 7 9 8 6 4 2

A CIP catalogue record for this book is available from
the British Library.

Phototypeset by Intype London Ltd
Printed and bound in Great Britain by
Mackays of Chatham plc, Chatham, Kent

With thanks to Ian, Keith, Sue, Helen, Jamie and Taryn for helping me survive my first year in practice, to Geoff Davis for all his advice and help at Vet School and to Tim Lawrence and family.

INTRODUCTION

This book is a diary of my first full year as a qualified veterinary surgeon. As you may know, through the BBC1 television series *Vets in Practice*, I qualified, along with my girlfriend Emma, from Bristol Vet School in the summer of 1996.

I decided to keep a diary of this year so that I could have a record of my experiences for later, to be able to look back at all the important cases and people which were probably going to influence my future career. I was once told that in the first year after leaving college you learn more than in the five years of training.

After my first year I think I agreed that nothing I had learnt at college could have quite prepared me for all the challenges which were to come my way in the following twelve months. Looking back, it was a great year, and I think I've come a long way. There were a few unpleasant moments, and the odd crisis but, all in all, it's been a very enjoyable start to my veterinary life.

This diary starts in January 1997, when I've been in my first job for a few months. The job is with a mixed country practice in Bideford, North Devon. Apart from myself, the new assistant, there are two other vets, Ian and Keith, who are equal partners in the practice. There are three veterinary nurses, Taryn, Helen and Jamie, and a receptionist, Sue.

Emma is working in Dulverton, Somerset, in a large-animal-orientated practice. It's about a forty-minute drive from Bideford, so we see each other most evenings.

The only other characters to introduce are Pan and Badger, our faithful dogs. When I first started work in Bideford, I decided that I could finally allow myself the luxury of owning a dog, after not having had one at home or college (my parents aren't doggy types, and university is no place to bring up a pet!). I heard of a litter of collie crosses on a farm nearby, and soon ended up bringing Pan home. The name came from a book I used to love as a child called *Bevis*, in which the hero, a young boy, has a faithful hound called Pan!

As soon as Emma saw Pan she decided that he would be much better off with some company, so the next day we went back to the farm and she picked one of his litter mates, Badger. I'm very glad we ended up having both of them; they're best mates.

January

Wednesday 1 January

9.00 a.m. Woken by phone from a deep hungover slumber. After spending the obligatory thirty seconds trying to turn off the alarm, and then realizing that it was in fact the phone, I finally spoke to an annoyingly cheerful Keith.

'Just giving you the phones,' he said. 'I'm off for a round of golf. Lovely day isn't it?'

What a wonderful start to the year: head throbbing, stomach churning and on call. At least I wasn't on call last night, although the way I feel right now I almost wish I had been.

9.17 a.m. First 'What time do you open this morning?' call. Very politely answered.

9.22 a.m. Second 'What time do you open this morning?' call. Still quite polite.

9.46 a.m. Third call. How can people expect me to a) know anything about, or b) be interested in, the dietary habits of their elderly hamster at this hour on New Year's Day? Not as polite. Must try and improve my telephone manner in these situations, after all hamsters are very important to some people.

9.57 a.m. Bloody hamster woman again. Must read up on causes of excess salivation in small rodents.

3 p.m. Hamster woman finally placated by a promise of a comprehensive dental examination tomorrow. I went down to Westward Ho! for some bread and milk, and walked Pan on the beach. He loves the sea and had a good swim even though the water is freezing. Last time I went surfing, a couple of days ago, it was too cold to be much fun. The surf was pretty good, but it's not the same trying to surf with a 5 mm wet suit, gloves, boots and a hat. Why can't I live in Hawaii?

I got back to find the answerphone flashing. I always

take the practice mobile out with me when I'm on call but it doesn't work very well down by the sea, so I have to be careful not to be out of contact for too long. The message was from David Gale, one of our best farm clients, who runs a large dairy herd a few miles out of Bideford.

'Er . . . um . . . this is David Gale, out at Lower Eastwood farm . . . er . . . we've got a cow in trouble, looks like she's brought her calf bed out . . . er . . . um . . . could you come out as soon as possible please?'

Resigning myself to missing breakfast (or lunch, as it was rapidly becoming), I headed off through town and out towards Torrington. Pan sat shivering on the back seat. I did try and warn him about the sea, but would he listen?

The cow had, as suspected by the farmer, pushed its womb out after calving. It was quite a nasty one to replace, I had to give her an epidural anaesthetic to stop her straining before I could gradually force the swollen mass of tissue back inside. Once it was finally in place, which took nearly an hour, I put in a couple of sutures to prevent a recurrence, and sank wearily on to a bale of straw. Most people would be lazing around at home after a nice lunch by now, but where was I? Sitting on a damp bale, covered in placental juices, aching and starting to shiver. Oh, what a great life it is being a vet!

At least the cow was OK, I suppose, and the farmer was really nice. Now I can go home, settle back, watch telly and relax for the rest of the day.

7.00 p.m. So far so good. Not even a phone call. Managed to watch the whole of *The Man with the Golden Gun* uninterrupted. Smell of placenta still refuses to budge from hands.

11.35 p.m. I spoke too soon. Just been called out to see a dog with diarrhoea. I should have told them to bring it in tomorrow, but they were pretty insistent I saw it tonight. I bet it's only mild colitis or something. Hardly a dire veterinary emergency.

Midnight Just as I suspected, mild colitis, which will clear up if they starve her (it was a lovely little spaniel bitch called Nesie). I gave her a couple of injections, to hasten her recovery, but I imagine she would have got over it pretty quickly anyway.

I've found in the time since I qualified last year that in many cases you end up treating the owners more than the animals. Quite often the animal will get better without any jabs or tablets, but the owner feels hard done by and cheated if they don't see something positive being done. At times, I think veterinary science is more psychology than medicine.

Thursday 2 January

6.00 p.m. Back at work today. I did morning surgery on my own as Keith had strained his back playing golf, and Ian had to go out to a calving first thing. It was pretty busy, lots of routine stuff, which is boring but doesn't require too much effort. At least they'd had the decency not to call me out yesterday to squeeze their dog's anal glands or clip their cat's claws.

Ian spent most of the rest of the day unblocking the drains at the back of the practice. He owns the building, so he has responsibility for its upkeep, although I would have thought that Keith, being twenty years younger, might have offered to help. I would have been straight in with the plunger, of course, but I was out on calls unfortunately! The practice is in an old Victorian house, set in about an acre of gardens, which is lovely but means that Ian seems to spend nearly as much time fixing things and mowing as he does consulting. He never complains though. I think he's one of these people who isn't happy unless he's busy.

Hamster woman came in with Jerry the hamster. I've always found hamsters quite hard to deal with; they tend to bite at the slightest provocation, or die as you try to treat them.

Jerry didn't die. He did, however, bite. As soon as I put my hand into his little box he latched on with all his might and refused to let go.

'Yes, he does nip occasionally when he's scared,' said hamster woman helpfully, as I resisted the overwhelming urge to bash Jerry on the side of the consulting table. 'I think it's his teeth that are the problem, don't you Mr Inglis?'

'Ahhh! Ouch! Yes, well, when he lets go, I'll be able to examine them,' I replied, applying a vice-like grip to his scruff and prising him off the remains of my index finger.

Jerry's front teeth were indeed overgrown, and were stopping him eating properly (although they didn't appear to be affecting his bite). A quick couple of clips and the problem was solved. I hope I'm not consulting next time his teeth need doing, I need my fingers for surgery.

There weren't any operations to do, so I had quite a quiet morning after surgery. This afternoon I had to visit a couple of clients, and then go and see a few lame cows. I managed to get out for half an hour before it got dark, and walk Pan down on the Northam Burrows. He's really growing fast now; he's going to be a big dog when he's fully grown. I hope Emma brings Badger over tonight, Pan really misses his brother when they're apart.

We keep saying we should take them back to the farm where we got them from to show the farmer how they are getting on. I'd like to see their mother again, she's a lovely big leggy farm collie. Their dad is a mystery, he's probably Tip, the nomadic crossbreed who wanders around Bradworthy and is reputed to have fathered most of the puppies in the area. Anne, a part-time vet at the practice, who lives near Bradworthy, told me Tip had recently been taken ill and may not be around to terrorize the local bitches much longer. I hope he's OK. He has what I feel is the perfect dog existence: roaming, shagging and eating – what a life!

10.35 p.m. Emma did come over, so we spent the evening

drinking wine and watching a video. Pan and Badger very happy.

Friday 3 January

11.00 p.m. Nothing too exciting happened today, just the usual mix of boosters, claw clips and off-colour dogs. Went to Jones's farm out at Hartland to do some fertility work with the scanner. I'm starting to get the hang of ultrasound scanning for pregnancy now I've been doing it for a few months. I'm pretty confident of getting it right from about thirty-five days of pregnancy onwards, although there are still cases where it's hard to be totally sure. I find it's best to be honest with the farmer when I'm doubtful and see the animal again a couple of weeks later, rather than guess and risk getting it wrong. It's not the same as in small-animal work where you can bluff your way through occasionally. Getting things like pregnancy diagnosis wrong can have very serious consequences for the farmer.

When I worked on a cattle station in Australia for a year before going to vet school I used to help the farmer pregnancy test his cows. The problem was that he could do it pretty well and I just used to feel inside and agree with him, without really having much of a clue as to *what* I was feeling. My downfall came when he asked me to check a cow he was going to shoot to eat (they used to get through a cow every three months or so).

'It's almost definitely barren,' he said, 'but just check anyway, would ya?'

I felt inside the cow. 'No, she's OK. No calf inside there,' I stated confidently. I couldn't admit to him that I wasn't entirely sure, so I decided he was almost certainly right and it would be best to agree with him.

The cow was then slaughtered and skinned. When we opened up the abdomen we found, to my horror, a large calf in the womb. This mistake on my part left the farmer several hundred dollars out of pocket, and me feeling awful not only about the farmer's loss, but also about the unnecessary death of the unborn calf.

Ever since then I've always been very cautious about pregnancy diagnosis in cattle, although I'm much more confident about my ability to know what I'm feeling for nowadays, and the scanner is excellent as you can actually see the foetus on the screen.

Saturday 4 January

3.00 p.m. I can't believe it! I'm on call this weekend. I thought Ian was on, but then he reminded me this morning that last month he had swapped a weekend with me. It's typical, there's some classic surf rolling in and I'm not going to be able to take advantage of it.

Ian's off to the AGM at Instow sailing club this evening, and he said that it's one of those boozy events which really isn't compatible with being on call. I can't imagine him racing single-handed dinghies in the sea, but he assures me that, come the summer, he'll be out on the water most weekends.

It's only six months since his heart bypass, but he looks fit as a fiddle and he's fully back at work now. He doesn't look like my idea of a typical heart-attack victim – he's lean and wiry with receding wild grey hair and amazing bushy grey eyebrows (not that bushy eyebrows are any indication of the health of one's heart!). He showed me the scar from his op the other day and it's amazing – a line all the way down his chest from top to bottom. It was such a shock when I arrived at the practice last summer to find out that he was in hospital for major heart surgery. He'd looked so well at my interview.

He's lived in Bideford for about thirty years, I think. Before that he worked somewhere up north in an old James Herriot-style farm practice. When he first started working here, the practice was based in a small terraced house next to the cattle market, and was run by a very eccentric old vet. They did probably 95 per cent large-animal work, only occasionally seeing a cat or dog. I think it's only been in the last ten years or so, since Keith arrived and the practice moved to Witten Lodge, that the small-animal side has started to grow. Ian's become really well known in the town as he's been the local vet for so long, and he's involved in the Rotary Club and things. I think he's taken over the mantle of eccentric old vet from his old boss!

Morning surgery was packed, we saw about twenty-five people, which is very busy for us. It gets quite tiring because it's an open surgery, so people keep wandering in just when you think you're nearly finished. Appointments are much better – at least you know how many people you've got to see and they don't all rush in together five minutes before the end.

I've just had to go and see a Labrador which keeps being sick. The owners, Mr and Mrs Johnson, are really nice. He kept referring to me as 'Doctor', which makes me feel very serious and important. The dog, a young black Lab called Jake, had been vomiting for a couple of hours when I arrived but wasn't looking too bad otherwise. His temperature was up a little and he had slight diarrhoea, but he seemed quite OK in himself. I suspected gastritis, so I gave him a couple of injections and suggested they starved him, but ensured he had plenty to drink.

Mrs Johnson was a little worried that Jake had eaten a plastic bag, and this might be causing his symptoms as she had seen him playing with one the night before. I told her I thought it was pretty unlikely, but said to call me if he didn't improve.

I hope it is just gastritis. It's always hard to know exactly what to do in situations like this because more than likely this is just a stomach upset, but there is a chance that it is a blockage. You have to take a sensible approach as you can't dive in and X-ray or open up every case. Hopefully, given twenty-four hours, he'll be fine and the plastic bag will turn up in the garden.

9.15 p.m. Mrs Johnson has just rung up to say that Jake has improved and has only been sick once since I left. This is good news, as it suggests my treatment is working and the possibility of a blockage is becoming less likely. He hasn't drunk much, though, but hopefully he will do overnight. Might consider putting him on a drip tomorrow if he still isn't drinking.

Sunday 5 January

Jake has taken a turn for the worse today. I was called round to see him again this morning and he had been sick again overnight. He still hadn't drunk enough fluids and was becoming quite seriously dehydrated.

I took him back up to the surgery and, with the help of one of the nurses, Helen, who lives above the practice, I put him on some intravenous fluids. We kept him at the surgery for most of the day while the fluids were slowly administered. By teatime he seemed much improved and brighter; he even managed a small drink and some liquidized food. I've sent him home on antibiotics and given Mrs Johnson some rehydration powders to mix up in his water to help replace the electrolytes he has lost by all the vomiting and diarrhoea.

I still think that it is a severe gastroenteritis, although a small voice inside me keeps reminding me that there could be a plastic bag blocking his gut which could rupture it. If I haven't got the diagnosis right, he could die.

If he's still bad tomorrow, we'll have him in and X-ray him. The owners seem like the type of clients who would rather spend the money on an unnecessary X-ray than risk losing their pet. People like this are so much nicer to deal with than the critical owners who question the cost of every treatment, and seem to expect you to come up with all the answers without spending any money or getting anything wrong. It always seems that you have to constantly balance what you would like to do for the animal against the cost to the owner and the likely outcome.

Monday 6 January

1.00 p.m. Just come home for some lunch after a hectic morning. Jake came back in looking awful. He'd been sick again through the night and was now very dull, depressed and dehydrated. Mrs Johnson was getting more and more concerned about him, and brought up the plastic bag theory again.

'I don't want to try and tell you what to do,' she said, 'but I'm really worried about him. I mean, shouldn't he be improving by now if it was just an infection? He seems so lifeless and – and I just want him to be all right.' She was almost in tears as she spoke, so I said we would keep Jake in this morning, put him on another drip, and take an X-ray of his abdomen. I still wasn't convinced that we would see anything, but the owner's distress meant we had to try and do something constructive. The little voice which was telling me I was wrong about the gastritis and that he did have an obstruction was getting harder to ignore.

We got him started on some fluids and then took a couple of X-rays. The practice hasn't got a developer yet so all the X-rays have to be taken up to the local hospital to be developed. This is a bit of a pain, but it can be quite useful as the staff are usually pretty interested in the pictures and help in interpreting the images. I looked at Jake's films half hoping to find evidence of a blockage so that we would at least have a definite diagnosis and could get on and treat him, but the pictures showed nothing conclusive. At vet school we were shown lots of classic X-rays of how intestines look with an obstruction, but out here in the real world of vetting nothing seems as clear-cut and simple as it is in textbooks and lectures.

I'm going to talk it over with Ian after lunch and see what he thinks. We may have to operate on Jake and have a look inside, we don't have many other options left.

7.00 p.m. I've just left Mrs Johnson at the surgery with Jake. He's coming round from his anaesthetic and she wanted to be with him as he wakes up. We finally took the plunge and opened him up at about four o'clock this afternoon. We decided we hadn't really got a choice, Ian didn't think he would make it through the night the way he was going.

Ian let me do the surgery, which was excellent as I've never done any major operations like this before. It all went really well. Once we'd knocked him out and stabilized him on some gas, I opened up his abdomen and found that all his small intestines were pleated together in a small tight ball. I incised the gut and pulled out a piece of plastic bag! Mrs Johnson had been right all along!

It took about half an hour and three incisions to get the whole bag out, and then even longer to suture the holes back together. It is really fiddly work and very tiring as you're concentrating so hard. It all looked OK, though, so his chances of pulling through should be reasonable. I just wish I'd listened to the owner instead of dismissing what she said so readily. She was so relieved and happy we had finally found out what the problem was she didn't even say, 'I told you so,' or, 'Why did it take you so long to realize what the problem was?' I wish all owners could be as nice and understanding as the Johnsons. They've been so good throughout and never once criticized what I was doing or got angry because he wasn't improving. They trusted my decisions although, in a way, it nearly cost them their dog.

10.30 p.m. Jake's looking excellent. He's up and about and has drunk a little water. I've told Mrs Johnson that although all is going well so far, he isn't out of the woods yet. There's still the risk of my sutures leaking, or peritonitis, or other complications. I really hope he's OK, I'd feel so guilty if he dies because I didn't operate soon enough, or because I did something wrong during the operation.

Was planning to go over to Dulverton to see Emma tonight, but I didn't want to leave Jake. Pan's been neglected today: only one decent walk. I think I'll take him out round the playing field for a run.

10.31 p.m. Raining, so let Pan into garden instead. Must stop being such a bad owner.

Tuesday 7 January

I couldn't sleep this morning as I was worrying about Jake. I got up and gave Pan a decent walk before going up to the surgery to check on Jake. I always dread the moment I first arrive when I have a critical case in the practice. I try my best to avoid all the nurses in case the news is bad, and usually rush out to the kennels and have a nervous glance at the animal before I see anyone.

My heart missed a beat or two when I first saw Jake lying, still, in his kennel, but as he heard me approach, he sat up and wagged his tail. I was very relieved!

Throughout the day he has improved dramatically, no more vomiting, and he is eating the liquid food we've given him. I really think he's going to be all right!

After sorting Jake out and ringing Mrs Johnson to keep her informed of his progress, I went out to a couple of farms. First I went to Mr Fulford's place on the other side of the river and saw a few fertility cases and a lame cow. Nothing too exciting except for Josie, the stockman's terrier, nearly getting kicked by one of the lame cows as I was trimming her hoof. Josie always hangs around the back end of the cattle crush eating all the nasty bits that I remove. I can't believe what dogs will eat – how any animal can find decaying placenta palatable is beyond me! Maybe Pedigree Chum should be made in three new exciting flavours – rotting flesh, hoof trimmings and clotted milk!

After Fulford's, I went on to Steve Thorne's out at Gammaton and saw some calves. They were in quite a state; coughing and not eating. It looks like pneumonia. I gave them all antibiotics and the worst ones a drug to bring down their temperature. I'm afraid he'll lose a few before we get the problem under control.

Emma came over from Dulverton again this evening because she finished earlier than me. I should make the effort to go over to her more, because she's always driving over here. We took the dogs up to the local for the first time and had a couple of pints and a few games of pool. They were really well behaved, apart from following me to the gents every time I went and Pan knocking over someone's drink with his tail. At least he didn't wee against the wall like he did in another pub.

Wednesday 8 January

Midnight, Dulverton Too drunk to write much, played in pool match in pub. Lost. Jake doing well.

Thursday 9 January

On call again. Jake went home today looking excellent. Mrs Johnson is so happy, and Mr Johnson said, 'Thank you, Doctor.' I wish we could call ourselves doctor, like vets do in America and the rest of Europe. Doctor Inglis sounds much better than Mr Inglis. Even dentists will soon be able to call themselves doctor, so if dentists (who, like doctors, all wanted to be vets but couldn't get the grades) can use that title I don't see why we shouldn't.

Quite a busy day at the surgery, lots of operations and

consulting. I did a bitch spay, two cat spays and a dog castration. I really enjoy surgery and doing the operation on Jake has boosted my confidence. Bitch spays are still a little nerve-racking though. Anne has been helping me by scrubbing up and holding things out of the way while talking me through the operation. The scariest part is breaking the ovarian ligament to free the ovary up so you can tie it off. You've got to be so careful not to pull too hard and rupture the blood vessels which lie right next to the ligament. So far all mine have been OK, but I've yet to do one completely on my own.

Only one call out so far tonight. I had to go out to Heard's farm out near Hartland for a calving. It was pretty straightforward so it didn't take too long, but I'm knackered after last night. I really hope I don't get called out again this evening, I could really do with a decent night's sleep.

Friday 10 January

8.00 a.m. Hooray! no calls.

8.07 a.m. Spoke too soon again. Mrs Johnson wants me to go and see Jake, she's worried about him. I'm really worried now. What if my sutures have come apart, or I left a bit of the bag in there somewhere? Damn! I so wanted him to be OK.

8.49 a.m. Jake is depressed again, but he's still eating and hasn't been sick. Mrs Johnson says he refuses to come out from under the coffee table, and is definitely not right. I checked his wound and it looks quite inflamed so, hopefully, he's just in a bit of discomfort from that and it's nothing more serious. Gave him a painkilling injection and said I would check on him later this evening.

Rest of the day was OK. Booked a bitch spay in to do solo in a couple of weeks. I hope I'm up to it. No farm work, so cleaned out the boot of my car. It was really starting to smell;

I think the bin full of dirty arm-length gloves didn't help. I got rid of the worst of it, but it's still a right mess. I think I may try and build a decent container for the boot to organize all my stuff and try to keep it in a reasonably clean state. Even Pan doesn't like the smell in the car, and that *is* saying something.

7.00 p.m. Jake much improved, and out from under the coffee table. I gave Mrs Johnson some painkilling tablets to give him over the weekend, and said we would take the stitches out as soon as possible next week as they are making his skin really sore.

Saturday 11 January

Worked until midday then off for the rest of the weekend. I had to go back and see Steve Thorne's calves after morning surgery. Two of the worst ones I saw on Tuesday have died and more are ill. He's been injecting them himself with antibiotic but it's not working, so I gave all of them a dose of a new antibiotic which is expensive but much more effective. He grumbled about the cost, but I reminded him that all the injections put together didn't even add up to the value of one calf. It's the best thing we've got to try and treat the disease, so if this fails he could stand to lose quite a few more calves. What he really needs to do is improve the ventilation in the calf-house. I think most farmers are under the misapprehension that pneumonia is caused by cold, so they block up all the windows and doors to keep the animals warm. In fact, that just makes things worse as warm stuffy places are prime sites for pneumonia to breed.

I always feel quite nervous when I'm telling farmers things like this as I'm only just qualified and they've been farming for years and years, so who am I to tell them what to do? What surprises me most is the way they do listen to what I'm saying, and respect my opinion – it's such a change from being a student when no one really takes much notice of anything you say.

Maybe I should grow a beard like Keith. I think farmers tend to see facial hair as a general indication of large-animal veterinary know-how! (All the best large-animal vets seem to have faces like overgrown gardens!) Saying that, I'm not sure that Keith really looks like a typical large-animal vet, he's a bit portly and too smart to quite look the part. His black hair and short beard are always a little too well groomed and his clothes too clean to give him that classic 'pulled through a hedge backwards' look of truly dedicated large-animal vets.

I think Ian and Keith are equal partners in the practice, although Keith only joined Ian about ten years ago. Veterinary partnerships are very complicated as far as I can see. When a new partner buys into the practice, they not only have to pay for their share of the physical assets, but also for things like goodwill and the client base. The more I think about it, the more I'm glad just to be the lowly assistant!

This afternoon I finally got to go surfing. Tim, my long-time surfing friend from university, came up from Bristol and we headed down the coast to a secluded reef break, which is near to some of our farms out at Hartland. When I first started here last summer I sometimes used to go to the coast after work if I was at a farm out this way. A few eyebrows were raised by some of the older farmers as I set off in the opposite direction to the surgery with my board in the car after finishing a line of pregnancy checks or lame cows.

We had an excellent surf, and then Tim, Emma and I went out into Bideford to a few pubs. Pan and Badger chewed the kitchen table while we were out. Mutts!

Sunday 12 January

Surf had dropped right off today so didn't go in. The beach is a right mess because a ship has dumped a load of tar out to sea which has washed ashore and left horrible sticky patches of black gunge all over the rocks. Badger got some on his paw and it wouldn't wash off and we ended up cutting the fur off. I trod some into the carpet so I've had to move the sofa to cover the stain. I hope Ian doesn't look under there if he checks the house over. The practice rents the house for me so if I trash it, they'll end up paying (or getting me to pay), which could cause a bit of tension at work. Getting a practice house is pretty standard for vets, and it makes a really nice change from living in horrible student flats at vet school.

I heard about the tar spillage on the radio this evening. Apparently several dogs have been burnt by it and people were told to contact their local vets if their pets eat any or get it stuck to them. I'm not quite sure what to do if a dog eats some caustic tar, I think I'd better read up my notes on poisons later on.

I played squash this evening up at Lenwood Country Club in Northam where I'm playing in a league. I thought my luck was in tonight because my opponent was about fifty and came on to court wearing two knee braces and a back support. Can't lose, I thought confidently, I'll just knock the ball around a bit, let him have a few points here and there and win comfortably. I lost 3-nil.

The evening turned out OK though, because over a beer in the bar afterwards I was telling my opponent about my grassboard invention and he turned out to be the boss of a local plastics company and said he could get me just the right material for the deck of the board. I've got some wheels and axles so once I get the deck I should be able to test the idea out – I hope it works, otherwise everyone who laughed at the idea will be right.

I first had the idea for a grass snowboard about two years ago, after I got back from a snowboarding holiday. I started to think that there must be a way of re-creating the sensation of snowboarding on grassy slopes. Over the next year or so I spent ages thinking about ways to make the board work and even made a few prototypes, including the infamous drainpipe and plywood disaster that made me the laughing stock of my friends in the fourth year at Bristol! I finally found inspiration while sitting in the bath at my mum's house in France. I suddenly worked out how I could get a board with wheels to work in the same way a snowboard does, by using a flexible deck suspended between two axles. The idea is that when the deck is leant, it forms an arc between the wheels, and the board steers in the same way that a snowboard bends and the board carves a turn through the snow. I really have high hopes that this idea will work. If it does, there is so much potential for the new sport to take off.

Monday 13 January

Late for work this morning because I locked the house keys inside when I took Pan out. It's been on the cards for ages. I really will get round to getting a second set of keys cut now. I had to ask next door if I could use their phone to ring Ian at the surgery. The people next door haven't liked me since I had a few friends round for the weekend last month and they all parked their cars in the communal car parking area. 'Each house is allotted two spaces and no more,' said the next-door neighbour. I thought he had a bit of cheek complaining after I'd squeezed his horrible poodle's anal glands last week free of charge. That's the last time I do him any favours.

Anyway, Ian eventually came round and let me in so I could get my car keys, and I was only about twenty minutes late for morning surgery. It was pretty busy, as it often is on a Monday, so we didn't finish until half-past ten. Afterwards, I had to go and see an ill dog. It turned out to be in the same little cul-de-sac that I live in, though it wasn't one of my near neighbours. The dog is fourteen and knackered. It can hardly get up because its hips are so arthritic and painful. I've put it on some anti-inflammatory drops but I think we'll have to put it to sleep before too long, which is a shame because the owner is obviously devoted to the old dog. I said I'd pop round and see how he was getting on after work tomorrow, but I can't see it really improving.

11.25 p.m. Bugger, forgot to get keys cut. MUST remember tomorrow!

Tuesday 14 January

1.00 p.m. Good morning – mainly farm work. Saw Steve Thorne's calves again, which are doing much better. One is still pretty ill so I gave him another shot of the new antibiotic, but the rest have responded very well. He hasn't done anything about improving the ventilation so I expect we'll see more problems in the next batch of calves put in the shed.

Mrs Johnson rang up to say that Jake was looking very well although his stitches were still irritating him. I've told her to bring him in tomorrow for stitches out.

11.10 p.m. What a terrible afternoon. It started badly because I had to do afternoon surgery, which was packed, when I was supposed to be operating on a dog with a bad eye. I really wanted to do the op but Keith decided he wanted to do it instead, so I ended up doing three boosters, a nail clip and two vaguely ill dogs. That got me in a bad mood, and then I had to go out to Brian Hill's farm near Hartland to see two lame cows, which is never any fun at the best of times.

It was tipping it down with rain, and a freezing wind was blowing in from the sea when I arrived. The farm is one of our less well-equipped and well-run places: nothing works, all the cows are covered in muck and they are nearly all lame. We tend to get called out only to the bad cases as Brian doesn't like spending money if the cows can still hobble around. These two were no exception, they were both severely lame in their back feet, and could hardly manage to limp into the rickety handling crush, which is very old and badly designed so that it's a real effort to get the cow in and restrained effectively. It is also outdoors so I got completely soaked.

The stockman, Graham, is OK. He at least cares about the cows, and does what he can to make the place better, but he's frustrated by Brian, who refuses to spend money on new facilities or the health of his cows. It really is disgraceful how badly farms can be run and still get away with it. I always hope that if I get reincarnated as a cow, I don't end up on a farm like this.

The first cow was the worst, its hoof was in a real state. A nail had penetrated the sole and set up an infection deep in the foot. This had spread underneath the sole, forming a foul abscess. I lanced it and then pared away all the areas where the infection had under-run the healthy sole, leaving the cow with just a small area of sound horn to walk on. It was a pretty gruesome job for me, and pretty painful for the cow, but it's her only real hope of survival. In most cases like this the cow doesn't get any local anaesthetic because it takes too long and by the time you've finished the injections, the job could have been done. It is nasty, but it's the way things are on farms. Most farmers wouldn't accept the need for a vet to give a time-consuming and expensive local anaesthetic block to a cow just to trim away an abscess. It's not that they don't care, it's just because they have to make a living from keeping animals. Some farmers definitely take this attitude too far, and treat their stock purely as money-making machines to be exploited, but most try to strike a balance between making a living and treating their animals well.

The other cow just had very overgrown feet, so she should do better, but she is still pretty lame. I wish we got called out earlier to cases like these, because then we might actually be able to do something for them, instead of trying to save an animal who is really beyond saving.

By the time I left I was soaking wet, freezing cold and smelling of cow muck and abscesses. Why do I do this job?

When I got home I soaked in the bath for half an hour and then went over to Dulverton. My hands still smell grim as I'm writing this. I may have to have them industrially steam cleaned.

Wednesday 15 January

6.45 p.m. Just finished evening surgery. The last appointment was an ancient old cat called Marmaduke. His owner was an equally ancient old woman called Mrs Thomas, who was very upset because she thought Marmaduke needed to be put to sleep. The cat was in a bad way: it had severe signs of kidney failure and a large ulcerated tumour on its lip. I asked her whether she thought Marmaduke had any quality of life left and she said no, all he did was sleep and he hadn't eaten for over a week. I told her I thought it would be the kindest thing, to put him to sleep, and she agreed, although it had obviously been a very hard decision for her to make.

Before I owned a dog, I never really appreciated how attached people can become to their pets and how upset they can get when it comes to times like this. Now I can really sympathize. If anything happened to Pan or he had to be put down, I would be devastated. I think all vets should own pets, because it does help you to understand how clients feel about their animals. I think it has helped me to help people through situations like the one confronting Mrs Thomas tonight.

The actual putting to sleep went smoothly, which is always a relief, especially when the owner is really upset. I always try to inject the drug into the vein, which is the quickest method, but sometimes you have to inject straight into the kidney in old cats. Marmaduke was lucky, he had good veins and didn't struggle, so it was all over in a matter of seconds.

When I was seeing practice, before I qualified, there was one awful vet who I really didn't like, because when he put cats to sleep he used to inject them in the abdomen and then leave the room while they went to sleep very slowly. He left the owners there on their own with their cat as it died, not explaining what he had done or what to expect. I think 95 per cent of vets really do care and try to do things properly, but there are definitely some around who seem not to care at all about animals. It makes me wonder why they became vets, because without a real love of animals I don't think anyone can be a good or happy vet. It's a bit like going into teaching if you hate children, I suppose.

9.26 p.m. Damn! Forgot to go round to see that old dog round the corner. Must remember tomorrow, and get some keys cut.

11.45 p.m. Had to go to a calving at 10 p.m. out at Paul Martin's farm. It was a real sod, the calf, coming backwards, dead and very smelly. Just going to have a bath in some bleach to get rid of the smell of rotting calf.

Thursday 16 January

Popped in to see the arthritic dog round the corner before work and it is much better on the drops, although it still has trouble getting up. The owner is very happy and wants to carry on with the treatment for now. Excellent.

Mrs Johnson brought Jake in to have his stitches out this morning (she couldn't make it yesterday). He looked so good, bouncing all over the consulting room, licking my face. He's a lovely dog. The stitches were really digging in, so he'll be very happy to have them out. I can't believe he survived! After all my messing about and waiting, then finally operating when it was nearly too late, he still pulled through. Mrs Johnson gave me a bottle of whisky for saving him, which is so nice of her. It's strange how you can almost make a real mess of a case but the animal survives and the owners are so grateful, when you can do everything by the book, and perfectly, and the owners complain and whinge and threaten to sue!

11.30 p.m. Whishky gon down vewy well, hic!

Friday 17 January

1.00 p.m. Finished for the weekend! Toby and Louise are coming up from Bridgewater for the weekend, which should be excellent. The surf isn't looking to good but it might get better tomorrow. I live in hope.

Surfing is like an addiction, because once you're hooked, you find yourself constantly thinking about it, and any decision has to include the thought 'will I be able to surf if I do that?' Ever since I joined the surf club in the first year at Bristol, I've spent my time either thinking about the last surf I had, or planning the next one. Even my choice of job was influenced by the fact that I wanted to be near the surf!

Monday 20 January

The weekend was great. On Friday we all went into Bideford and got pissed, then went for a curry. On Saturday, after recovering with a massive fry-up, went surfing over at Croyde. The surf was pretty good, about four feet and clean, but it was absolutely freezing. The wind was howling off-shore from the east, which made it really hard to get down the front of the waves without being blown off backwards.

Emma and Louise have started surfing (well, Louise is boogie-boarding, which doesn't really count – lying on a half-size foam board on your stomach isn't quite the same as standing up on a proper surf board) and got on pretty well. Afterwards we went to the pub to thaw out. We were so cold that we ended up actually putting our feet in the gas fire to try to regain some feeling. Emma was the shade of blue usually only seen in dogs about to die from heart failure!

On Sunday we went for a long walk along the coast path with the dogs as the surf had dropped right off. I saw loads of potential grassboarding slopes to try out once the first prototype is finished. Toby has no faith in the idea at all, he thinks I'll break either my legs or my head on the way down. I'll show him! He'll be laughing on the other side of his face when the grassboarding empire takes off and I'm a millionaire! Well, I can dream I suppose – I'm never going to be a millionaire by being a vet, that's for sure.

Today was pretty unexciting, lots of boosters and non-pregnant cows. After work I went to B & Q and bought some bolts and springs to build the first grassboard prototype. I spent most of the evening in the spare room drilling and sawing away (much to Emma's delight!) and I think I've got something which could work. I'll try it out tomorrow.

Emma's very patient with me most of the time, and doesn't get too annoyed when I spend an entire evening working away on some project or other. I suppose she's got used to it over the eighteen months we've been seeing each other, since the beginning of the final year of vet school.

Tuesday 21 January

1.30 p.m. Did my first solo bitch spay today. It was a nice easy little terrier and everything seemed to go pretty well. I kept checking her colour every five minutes after the op to make sure she wasn't bleeding inside and, so far, it all looks OK.

6.15 p.m. Bitch spay went home looking good, so nothing should go wrong now. I'm still half convinced that I'll get into work tomorrow and Ian will tell me that he was called out to see her in the middle of the night and she bled to death. I must stop worrying so much about operations.

I had an hour off this afternoon so I took the MkI grassboard out for its first trial run on a small hill near the practice – and it worked! Well it kind of worked, anyway. It turned and went OK but I kept falling off and it was very hard to control. My work trousers are covered in grass stains and I ripped my shirt but, apart from that, no serious injuries! I think it needs some more development before I can release it on the public!

Wednesday 22 January

7.00 p.m. On call tonight. Today was quite good, lots of appreciative owners and nice pets. A woman brought in a couple of geese. We had to inject them against worms, which was OK until one of them decided to crap all over my white coat and trousers. It amazed me quite how much mess an average goose could produce.

7.45 p.m. Just starting dinner, called out to see a dog. Sounds like a possible gastric torsion, which could be interesting. Better hurry.

1.15 a.m. I am exhausted! I've just spent the last two hours operating on this dog, and I still think it may die. It was a gastric torsion, where the stomach twists round and becomes filled with gas, which I had suspected from what the owner told me over the phone.

'He's been bringing up white froth for the last hour and his tummy looks ever so swollen,' she'd said in a state of panic.

As soon as I saw the dog, an elderly boxer called Rufus, my suspicions were confirmed. His belly was rock hard and about twice its normal size. He couldn't walk, so his owner,

Mrs Cave, carried him into the consulting room and laid him on the table. He was so weak he couldn't even lift his head up when I approached him.

'I'm afraid Rufus has a twisted stomach,' I told Mrs Cave, once I had examined him. 'It's a very serious condition, and he may not pull through. We'll do what we can, though. Firstly I'm going to put him on a drip, then we'll try to deflate his stomach.'

There were no nurses around so I had to ask Mrs Cave to help me put the drip in, which she managed very well considering the circumstances. Once we had fluids going in, I tried to pass a stomach tube, but I couldn't get it down because of the twist in the stomach. Rufus was looking really grim by now, his colour was awful and he was getting weaker by the minute, so I decided to try to deflate his stomach by putting needles into it, through his flank. He didn't flinch as I passed a large needle through his skin and into the swollen organ below. As the needle pierced his stomach a hiss of escaping gas was emitted and the swelling gradually started to subside. I put in four or five more needles to hasten the process.

'That should ease the swelling and buy us some time, but it won't really solve the problem,' I said. 'Once he's had some fluids and his colour has improved, I'll have to operate to untwist the stomach otherwise the swelling will return, and if that goes on for too long, his stomach will become over-stretched and the tissue will die. If that happens, his chances are very poor.'

I also told her that I would need some help with the operation and I was going to call out one of the other vets. I rang Ian and, although he was in the middle of a dinner party, he promised to come down as soon as I was ready to operate.

Mrs Cave decided to go home and await the outcome there, so I sat alone with Rufus in one of the kennels for an hour while the fluids dripped in. At about eleven I called Ian again and he came down to help.

We thought it best to operate immediately as his chances of making it through the night were slim, so we knocked him out and tried to do our best to save him, although we both knew that the odds were stacked against him.

As soon as we opened the abdomen we knew things were very bad. Part of his stomach was a dark reddish-black colour and his spleen was grossly engorged, suggesting the torsion had been present for longer than the owner had thought. Over the next two hours we managed to untwist the stomach and decompress it via a stomach tube, and remove his spleen, which had also been twisted along with the stomach. Then we sutured the stomach to the muscle of the body wall to stop it re-twisting, and finally stitched him up and took him off the gas.

He was looking reasonable when we eventually left a few minutes ago, but I'm very worried about the state of his stomach wall. If the tissue doesn't recover from not having any blood supply while it was twisted, he won't make it.

Thursday 23 January

He didn't make it.

I arrived in a state of nervous excitement as usual when cases like this are in, knowing that he probably hadn't survived, but with a little glimmer of hope that he would be up and wagging his tail. I was so disappointed when I went to the kennel and found the nurse cleaning it out, with Rufus's body lying in a black bag on the floor.

'He didn't survive then,' I said pointlessly to Helen. 'I thought he wouldn't, but it's still such a shame. I wonder if we should have done something different, maybe we shouldn't have operated so soon, I don't know.'

'Don't worry about it too much,' replied Helen. 'I've seen loads of torsions since I've been here, and only one or two have survived.' It was nice of her to try and make me feel better but I still felt pretty bad that I'd been unable to save him.

Mrs Cave was all right about it. I think she was expecting bad news because she didn't seem too surprised when I told her what had happened. She wants him to be individually cremated so she can have his ashes back and scatter them on the Northam Burrows, where she always used to walk him.

The rest of today was fairly quiet; one farm visit to see an ill cow and sign a couple of slaughter certificates and afternoon surgery. Emma came over this evening and I told her all about Rufus. She said that she would have done exactly the same things as I'd done, which is good to know. It is so nice seeing someone who is also a vet so we can talk over things like this.

Friday 24 January

Much better day today, no more deaths or difficult cases, just lots of nice straightforward lame dogs, cats with abscesses and rabbits with overgrown teeth.

I had a call from someone at the BBC. Apparently they want to film me and Emma for the follow-up series to *Vet's School*, which will be excellent. They're coming down next week to take us out for lunch and explain what they want to do. I hope it works out, I'd love to be on TV!

Saturday 25 January

1.00 p.m. Home for lunch. Morning surgery was packed, as it usually is on a Saturday. After Ian and I had finished, I had to go out to Brown's farm and see a cow that had trodden on one of its teats. It was a real mess and very awkward because the cow kept kicking me as I tried to stitch the wound. After getting a nasty kick on the arm and swearing at the cow a lot, I eventually managed to cobble the lacerated teat back together. I'm not convinced that it'll heal very well, because it was such a nasty cut and the milk tends to stop the tissues joining together. I've only seen one other case like this, which was much easier because the cow also had milk fever so it was lying down in a field. This meant I could stitch it up without having to dodge flying hooves, and once I'd finished I gave her some calcium to treat the milk fever so she could get up. She went on to do very well, but I think that she was the exception rather than the rule in these cases.

When I got back to the surgery Ian said, 'Why didn't you give her a sedative?' and I wondered why I hadn't thought of that. It's strange how in stressful situations you can completely forget to think logically or use your commonsense. If I had only stopped to think instead of getting angry and shouting at the poor cow I could have saved myself a lot of pain and aggravation.

I was quite lucky not to have been hurt. Cows' hooves can cause some serious damage, although saying that, I've been injured more often by small animals than farm animals, especially cats and, of course, the most fiercesome of them all, the dreaded hamster! I'm sure that more vets have been injured by hamster's teeth than cows' hooves or cats' claws.

I'm on call all weekend, but at least there's no surf. There is nothing more frustrating than seeing lovely surf but not being able to go in because you're on call. Once, last year, I was so keen to go in that I paid one of the nurses to take the phones for me while I went surfing, and told her to come and wave at me from the beach if I was urgently needed. Luckily there weren't any calls.

I think I'll try the grassboard out some more this afternoon, I can transfer the calls to the mobile and carry that with me while I cruise down the hills.

4.00 p.m. All was going fine until two things happened. Firstly, the MkI grassboard failed to negotiate a small tree stump and is now in several pieces and secondly, as I was lying on the ground nursing a bruised elbow, the phone rang and I had to go to see a cow with milk fever out at Mr Chamings' farm. I don't think he was too impressed when I turned up in a pair of grass-stained overalls and large muddy snowboarding boots!

It was quite an advanced case; the cow was wedged in a cubicle and couldn't get up. The farmer had already given her a calcium injection under the skin but when she still didn't get up, he called me to give her some intravenously. Luckily I got the vein first time, which is always a relief because I feel that farmers tend to judge you initially by how well you can do simple things like i/v injections. If you can't even get a vein then they think you're not going to be any good at more complex stuff, which is probably a fair assumption. One of my predecessors had quite a bad reputation among a lot of the farmers because she often had to call out one of the partners to help her do i/v injections in cattle. The farmers saw this as a fairly basic failing and therefore didn't have confidence in her abilities to do other things.

Anyway, once the cow had had a bottle of calcium intravenously, she immediately stood up and walked out of the cubicle with nothing worse than a scuffed hip to show for her ordeal. It's always one of my favourite moments in being a vet, seeing cows stand up so quickly after treating milk fever. One minute they are helplessly stranded, lying on the ground slowly dying and then, literally seconds after you've treated them, they get up and walk away – I wish all my patients could be cured as simply as that!

I think I'll have to take the grassboard to an engineer to get a more sturdy prototype made, the MkI is definitely beyond repair.

Sunday 26 January

11.00 p.m. A very lazy day today, no call outs at all, which is amazing (mustn't speak too soon though). Emma was on call this weekend as well, which means we haven't seen each other since Friday, but at least we'll have a weekend off together next week.

I took Pan for a walk on the beach this afternoon. The surf is still as flat as a pancake thankfully, although there were still a few desperate people out there trying to surf the six-inch ripples that were rolling in. I used to be the same when I was at university in Bristol. You would drive all the way down to go surfing at the weekend only to find that the promised five-foot classic swell had mysteriously dropped off to one-foot rubbish, but you felt you still had to go in because you had driven so far to get here.

Pan picked up a rotten fish on the beach and was most upset when I made him leave it. Quite what attraction he sees in a piece of half-chewed, foul-smelling fish is beyond me, although he tried to persuade me by licking my face immediately after dropping the fish!

Emma rang up earlier and said she'd had a really busy weekend. On Saturday she saw three calves with pneumonia, a calving and a horse with a cut leg, and today she's been out to about four different farms for various things. She tends to see completely different cases to me because most of the farms around Exmoor are small basic beef and sheep farms, whereas around here they are mainly large well-run dairy farms. She also deals with the hunt a lot, treating the horses and hounds, as stag hunting is a very big part of community life around Dulverton. Emma is very anti-hunting because she feels it is cruel both to the stags and to the hunting horses and hounds. I don't like the cruel part of it, and I wouldn't take part myself, but I believe people have a right to do it and that it is an integral part of country life in areas like Exmoor. If hunting was banned, I think country communities would suffer enormously, and that would include country practices like Emma's, which rely heavily on work generated by hunting.

I must stop rambling on about things like this just before I'm going to bed, I'll never get to sleep now.

Monday 27 January

6.00 p.m. Had to rush out to Lake's farm this morning before surgery to see a cow which had started bleeding as it tried to calve. When I arrived there was a large pool of blood spreading behind the recumbent cow, and just one of the calf's legs visible. I felt inside, but I couldn't tell where the blood was coming from because the calf was in the way, so I quickly pulled its other leg into position and eased it out as gently as possible. As soon as it was out of the way, I could feel the end of a large artery pumping blood from the wall of the vagina. After a few minutes of groping around, I managed to apply a pair of clamps to the blood vessel and the flow of blood was stemmed. I tied the handle of the clamps to the cow's tail so that if they were dislodged, they wouldn't disappear (inside or outside of the cow), and then inserted one of the farmer's finest bath towels to form a plug and help prevent any further bleeding.

She looked OK when I left, although she was weak from loss of blood and the effort of calving. I think I probably looked worse actually, because I was covered in blood and slime. I had to nip home and change before morning surgery. I thought I had washed all the blood off, but as I was having a cup of coffee after surgery, one of the nurses pointed out a large blob of congealed blood in my hair. No wonder I had been getting such funny looks from clients all morning!

After that early excitement, the rest of the day was pretty quiet, just a few routine ops, one farm visit, and a nearly empty afternoon surgery. The BBC rang again, and they want to try a day's filming on Thursday.

Midnight, Dulverton Pub, pool and too much Guinness. Pan has developed a very strange fixation with the dart board. He now runs in and sits under the board all night, staring up at it as if he's guarding his master's grave. He's had a few very near misses with stray darts. I'm sure he'll end up with one embedded somewhere and we'll have to rush him down to the practice for emergency dart-removal surgery. Dogs really are very odd creatures!

Tuesday 28 January

Took the grassboard into a small engineering firm in Bideford today and asked if they could build me a sturdier version. Peter Bullock, who runs the firm (in fact I think it is a one-man firm), seemed to think that it shouldn't be a problem. He didn't look at me as if I was stark raving mad, which was nice. I think he has to deal with quite a few eccentric inventors so he's probably used to people coming in with weird and wonderful contraptions. The only real problem is sorting out how to get the springs to work properly. He thinks that rubber bushes would be better, but I'm not convinced, so I've asked him to build it with springs for now and we'll see how it comes on.

I had a very busy morning out pregnancy testing with the ultra-sound scanner. I did about forty cows in one stint at Charles Moore's farm. I like going out there, everything is well organized and they really make an effort to look after their cows. I think this repays him, as healthy cows perform better and preventive medicine is always cheaper than curative treatment. Charles is into homoeopathic medicines for his calves and, although I'm a bit sceptical, they certainly seem pretty healthy at the moment.

It's very hard to believe in alternative medicines such as

homoeopathy when you've just spent five years at university having conventional theory drilled into you, because it often goes completely against the basic scientific rules that you've been taught, but when you actually see them working they become harder and harder to discount. Acupuncture I find much easier to believe in, as I can see how pressure in certain specific points could trigger various chemical/hormonal releases which would affect other parts of the body. I've not seen it done myself, but one of my friends who is working in a practice in Leeds says it can have amazing results in cases such as arthritis in dogs. Maybe one day I'll look into it a bit more. I think not giving alternative treatments a chance is very short-sighted as, if they weren't at least partially effective, why would oriental medicine for humans be based on these techniques?

While we were scanning Charles's cows for pregnancy, I found one with a very strange, large mass on her right ovary. It was much bigger that a cyst, which are quite common, and was solid and very uneven in texture. I told Charles I thought it was an ovarian tumour and that there wasn't an awful lot we could do about it. In a dog or cat we would have a go at removing it but, although it may be technically possible, it's just not economically viable to attempt such an operation in a cow. Most of the few operations done on cattle in this country are caesareans and operations to correct displaced stomachs. Both are relatively simple and cheap to perform. In Australia, the farmer I worked for used to spay cows to stop them getting pregnant so they could be fattened up. The operation was performed with no anaesthetic and very basic hygiene standards and, as a result, about one in twenty died. This was acceptable there, though, as cows were worth so much less than in this country and the whole mentality behind what was and wasn't acceptable to do to animals was completely different. Some of the things that went on in Oz made hunting stags look like a quiet, kind walk in the country.

Wednesday 29 January

10.30 p.m. On call tonight. Had to go and see a cat for someone up in Northam which turned out to be dead (and stiff) when I arrived. Apparently the woman had seen it jump off the garden wall on to the drive and it hadn't moved. It wasn't her cat so she hadn't been too worried, but now she wanted to get her car out and didn't want to touch it or move it. It had been dead for several hours by the time I arrived, so all I did was pick it up and take it away. After she gets the bill I think the woman will find she overcomes her dislike of touching dead animals in the future!

Thursday 30 January

8.15 a.m. BBC are here today, must look smart and suitably vet-like.

8.17 a.m. Damn! Just found best work trousers underneath pile of dirty washing, still covered in blood from the other morning. I'll have to wear reserve pair.

8.20 a.m. Reserve trousers split in crotch, disaster!

8.25 a.m. Finally had to resort to reserve pair two, which are too short, have no button, and a very suspicious stain on the left thigh. I think I'll try and see if the BBC can avoid any detailed trouser shots and concentrate on my clean and ironed shirt.

1.00 p.m. Well, that was a very stressful morning. The BBC were there waiting for me when I arrived and then got straight on with filming morning surgery. There were four of them, a director called Sarah, a researcher called Emma and a cameraman and a soundman, both called John, I think. They all seemed very nice and did their best to put me at ease, but it was still quite daunting having a massive camera and sound boom hovering around in the consultation. I was pretty nervous to begin with, and was looking at the camera too much and not concentrating on the animals (I came very close to giving a cat a dog booster!). After a while, though, I got a bit more used to it, and I think they started to get some usable footage.

The most interesting case they filmed was a basset-hound called Hobo who came in with his owner, an oldish lady called Mrs Hartley. Hobo had a bad ear, and every time Mrs Hartley had tried to clean it out, Hobo had bitten her on the arm. She showed me the scars and bruises on her forearm, which made me a little cautious about having a look in his ears myself. He was pretty well behaved while I examined him, and didn't even object as I gave his ears a gentle clean and applied some medicated drops – maybe he knew that the cameras were there and didn't want to look like a villain on TV! Anyway, I told Mrs Hartley to bring him back every day for a week or so and we'd clean them and apply the drops to see if we could cure the problem – without her losing her arm.

7.00 p.m. Very tired. It's been a long stressful day, but enjoyable as well. The BBC reckon they got some good material today and said they would like to come back next week to do a few days on the trot. I said yes, mainly because I hope I'll get some more delicious pub lunches out of them. I mentioned the grassboard and they seemed quite interested, so hopefully they'll film it and the publicity will help launch the idea. Either that or the entire nation will think I'm mad!

Friday 31 January

Emma's Birthday

11.30 p.m. Dulverton Just got in from the pub, after having a lovely meal at a local restaurant. I bought Emma some CDs and some wetsuit gloves and boots so that she has no excuse not to come surfing. She seemed to like the CDs more than the surfing stuff, for some reason. I think deep down she doesn't really want to try surfing and is only pretending to be enthusiastic for my sake. Never mind, at least she can't say that I haven't tried to get her into it.

I can't really remember what I did at work today, too much wine and Guinness, I think, but I'm off for the rest of the weekend, so I can relax and have a lie in for once.

February

Monday 3 February

8.20 a.m. Dulverton Damn!

8.55 a.m. Bideford Only ten minutes late, but I'm still the first vet here.

1.00 p.m. I can't believe I overslept this morning, it's lucky that Pan and Badger decided to come and jump on the bed when they did, otherwise I could still be snoozing away in Dulverton! The weekend was excellent, I actually got Emma to try a bit of surfing and she really enjoyed it (apart from getting held under by a big wave, which scared her a bit). On Sunday we took the dogs for a decent walk up on Exmoor, which was fun until the mist came down and we nearly got lost on top of the moor. The dogs were useless at finding our way back to the car, they just kept chasing each other and barking at bushes.

This morning has been hectic, which was the last thing I needed on a Monday. After morning surgery I had four farm calls all at different corners of the practice, so I've spent most of my time in the car and very little actually treating animals. My car, or rather the practice's car, which I use, is beginning to suffer from too many farm tracks driven too fast. I took it to a jet wash last week to try and clean the outside, but even the high-pressure hose failed to move some of the really ingrained stains. White is a silly colour for a vet's car anyway!

9.00 p.m. On call this evening because Keith is off this week. Mrs Hartley came in for me to clean Hobo's ears again. They were still very infected and sore, and I got lots of wax and muck out of them. He wasn't quite so well behaved without the cameras there, and we had to put a muzzle on him to stop him snapping.

Mrs Hartley seems very grateful for what we are doing – I think I'm a bit of a soft touch when it comes to helping people out who can't really afford the treatment. She's promised to pay us what she can every week, and I'm trying to keep the bill as low as possible, but it's still mounting up. I feel quite sorry for her because, although Hobo can be a bit nasty at times, she obviously loves him and he's all she's got. Some older vets tend to get a bit cynical about cases like this, which I suppose comes when it's your money that is being spent not the bosses'. I hope that if I become a partner I don't always let money rule in cases like this because, in a way, it's people like Mrs Hartley and animals like Hobo who need treatment the most, and just because they haven't got lots of money doesn't mean they don't deserve our attention. I know that vets have to earn a living, but I think there should always be room for a little leeway in some cases.

I've told Mrs Hartley not to mention all the daily ear-cleaning sessions to Ian or Keith!

Tuesday 4 February

6.00 p.m. Good easy day today. Morning surgery was almost empty, Ian and I only saw three people between us, and two of those were post-op checks. After sitting around reading the *Vet Record* and drinking tea for the best part of an hour, I went out to disbud and castrate a few calves.

I quite enjoy castrating and disbudding, as long as there aren't too many to do at once. Disbudding involves removing the horn buds from young calves using a red-hot iron. Although this is one instance where local anaesthetic is routinely used, it's still pretty unpleasant for the calves. It can be hard work physically, but it gives you a chance to work on automatic pilot while you chat to the farmer. I like talking to farmers because you can be yourself and don't have to worry about being too polite or tactful. It makes a change from small-animal work, where you're always having to put on a cheerful, respectable face and trying to be polite and sensitive. Farmers tend to appreciate less censored conversation and don't object to swear words or the odd rude joke.

Emma, from the BBC, rang up this afternoon and asked if they could come and film next week. I hope we have some interesting cases for them. I feel a bit under pressure to produce some good exciting stories, otherwise they won't want to come back and film again. Maybe there'll be a decent cow caesar or another gastric torsion (but preferably one that survives).

Wednesday 5 February

On call again tonight thanks to Keith being off. He and his wife have gone to Egypt for a week's cruise on the Nile – it's a good life being a partner!

I had a big scanning session out at Charles Moore's farm this morning. I did over forty cows, which took about two hours. I can hardly move my left arm now!

I got chatting to Charles about how his farm was progressing and the difficulties he was having. He mentioned that he was going to a meeting next month about problems associated with incorrect feeding of cattle and how it affects fertility and he's offered to take me along as he thinks his vet should know a bit more about things like this. It sounds quite useful because, although we learned a lot about nutrition and fertility at university, I've just about forgotten it all now, and I'd like to be able to give better advice to farmers about feeding because it's really the most vital part of raising cattle well.

Some large-animal vets are moving more and more towards becoming just nutrition and health advisors rather than actually treating sick animals. Prevention of diseases and health problems is always better than treating them when they happen.

I saw a practice in Salisbury before I qualified where

there were three vets who did nothing except large-animal work, and they told me they could see that in five years or so they would do virtually no 'fire-brigade' work (emergencies, etc.), but concentrate instead on advising farmers on feeding and general husbandry. I thought at the time that this was all very well and probably is the future of large-animal vetting, but where was the excitement and enjoyment in doing work like that?

I still feel I would get pretty bored just advising farmers on protein ratios and ventilation rates, but since I've been in practice I can definitely see the attraction in doing some work like that. It would be very satisfying to prevent mass health problems or increase the farmer's productivity by simply advising him on where he was going wrong.

At present I feel I can offer some useful advice, but I don't really know enough to be very helpful. I can remember bits of what we were taught but I tend to get halfway through telling a farmer how he needs to change his calf feeding programme and then realize I can't quite remember exactly the details of the correct way to do it. This either means that I have to bluff my way through, which is a dangerous game with farmers, or admit my failure and risk losing credibility.

I'm going to ask Ian if I can go to this talk, and I'm also going to try and make myself re-read my old notes.

I can't believe how much I've forgotten in the six months since I qualified. When I took my final exams last June, I knew so much, and now it seems that all that hard-learnt information is gradually disappearing. I suppose that although I don't know nearly as much detailed theory as I did six months ago, I'm replacing it with new, more relevant, knowledge gained from clinical experience rather than studying textbooks. Sometimes, though, when I have for-gotten something and I look it up in a book, it's amazing how the old knowledge comes back. Presumably once it's been learnt it never actually goes away, it's just filed in some deep, obscure place in the murky mists of the brain!

I think my knowledge is shifting from a broad, theoretical mass of information to become more specific and useful, and more based on clinical experience than textbook theory. Sometimes I wonder whether all the irrelevant information we are taught at vet school is really worth learning, but I suppose that, because vets do so many different and varied jobs, the teaching has to be very wide ranging. Once we qualify, it's up to the individual vet to select what is relevant to them and build on that with clinical experience.

Thursday 6 February

8.30 p.m. Knackered! I was up until about 2 a.m. last night doing a horrible calving. I got called at about 10 p.m. and drove over to this farm, which I'd never been to before, on the other side of Barnstaple. It took me a while to find the place because it was down a small track in between some houses on the edge of town, so I didn't arrive until gone half past.

The farm was one of the few really small old-fashioned farms left in the area. Most of our farms are pretty big and modern, usually having between seventy and two hundred cows, but there are still a few little places around which have hardly changed for years, with twenty or thirty cows and really basic facilities. The farmers tend to be really nice and hospitable, but it's still frustrating going to these farms because the animals are often kept in a pretty awful state.

This place was fairly typical of this type of farm. The farmer had about thirty-five dairy cows which were housed in an ancient set of cow kennels. Kennels differ from more modern cow-houses in that the stalls where the cows lie support the roof directly rather than having separate stalls in a large free-standing shed. In this case there were two rows of kennels facing each other, separated by a roofless passage where the cows dunged.

The stalls where the cows could lie were in a pretty grim

45

state, with minimal bedding and lots of muck everywhere. It was pouring down with rain when I arrived, and because the cow which was calving was in one of the stalls, I had to kneel down in the exposed passageway to try and calve her, with a foot of slurry under me and rain soaking me as it poured off the kennel roofs.

There were no lights, so the farmer had to park his battered old Land-Rover in the passage to light up the area. At this point I really thought things were about as bad as it gets, I was freezing cold, covered in muck and breathing in choking diesel fumes. However, when the farmer's son arrived with a bucket half full of absolutely icy cold water I realized things could indeed get worse!

The cow was lying on her side, wedged in the stall. Apparently she'd started calving the night before, and had been lying there, straining in the muck, for over twenty-four hours. I felt inside, and found one of the calf's front feet and its nose. I put a rope around the leg, and managed to get another round the head. Then I felt inside for the other front foot, eventually found it and, after a lot of struggling and swearing, brought it up and got a rope on it. Now I was in a position to start pulling, so I gave the farmer and his son a rope each and felt inside as they started to pull. I could feel the calf start to come a little, but then it stopped and refused to move any further.

The problem was obvious – the calf was too big for the cow's pelvis. It was also swollen and dry after being squeezed by its mother for the last twenty-four hours. I decided to put loads of lubricant around the calf to see if I could gradually ease it out using the calving jack.

I fetched the calving jack from my car and assembled it. It looks like an instrument of torture from the Middle Ages, designed to pull people apart, but it is really useful in tight calvings like this. It's basically a ratchet system which pushes against the back of the cow while pulling on the calving ropes attached to the calf inside.

With the jack attached to the ropes, I asked the farmer to apply pressure gradually while I added more lubricant and tried to guide the calf out. It was no good, though, the calf wasn't moving, and I was worried about using too much force in case I damaged the calf or the cow.

I spent the next forty minutes desperately trying to manoeuvre the calf so it would move, but with no luck. All the time I was lying there, wrestling inside the cow, I was getting more and more worried about what I was going to do next. I could try and do a caesarean but the chances of it being successful, with a calf that was probably dead and in a filthy cow cubicle with poor light, were slim. It would also be my first solo cow caesar. The other option was to try and cut up the calf in situ and bring it out bit by bit, but I wasn't even sure that it was dead, let alone that I had the necessary equipment in the car to do an embryotomy.

In the end, I had to admit defeat and tell the farmer I was going to call Ian out to help. I felt pretty bad, but I thought it was the best thing for everyone, including the cow. I rang Ian, and he said that he would come straight over.

It took him about forty-five minutes to get there (he said he'd had to take the back road as he'd had quite a lot of wine that evening). During this time I sat in the farmer's kitchen and chatted to the farmer and his wife. They seemed pretty understanding about it all, but it must have been annoying for them because it was now getting on for 1 a.m.

When Ian arrived he was really good about it, and said it was quite normal to need help on the occasional hard calving. This made me feel better, but I knew that he must have been pretty pissed off to have to come all the way out on his night off.

At this point, I was really hoping that Ian wouldn't just reach in and pull out the calf straight away. He didn't, but he did succeed after about twenty minutes, pulling out a very dead and battered calf. He had felt inside and decided that the only option was to pull the calf out in one piece. He ended up having to use two calving jacks to apply enough force to get the calf out, gradually applying more and more pressure until the shoulders were forced out and then the rest came relatively easily.

Although he'd succeeded where I had failed, I felt I had been right in what I'd done. I'd been unable to get the calf out because I'd not pulled hard enough, but after seeing the calf being winched out with two calving jacks applying literally tonnes of force, I thought it may have been better not to have bothered, and to have shot the cow. It seemed inhumane and cruel to me to put an animal through such intense suffering, I really believed I had been justified in stopping when I had, and that I should have had the confidence to tell the farmer the cow should be destroyed.

Ian comes from an era of vets who are more used to treating animals in this way – it was the norm a few years ago. It isn't a lack of care or skill or anything on his part, it's just a different way of thinking.

When we left, at about 2 a.m., the cow was still lying in the passage. I think because the calving was so tight, it may have damaged some nerves and she may never recover.

Today, I went back and saw the cow again. She was still down, despite having calcium and a painkiller, so I suspect that after all our efforts last night, she is not going to survive. I feel bad for the cow, because of what she suffered, and bad for the farmer because he's spent quite a lot of money on vets' fees and has ended up with no calf and probably no cow. For a small farm such as this, with only fifty or sixty cows in the herd, the loss of one milking cow and a potential replacement in the calf can be a serious blow.

This case has taught me a few things. I think I need to have more confidence in my skill and stick to what I feel is the right thing to do, rather than assume that I'm wrong and pass the decision on to someone else, who may end up doing something which I don't really agree with.

Friday 7 February

1.30 p.m. Mrs Hartley came back in this morning with Hobo. His ears are better but still really inflamed and sore. I've told Mrs Hartley that I think the best thing would be to do an aural resection, designed to open up the ear canal to let all the infection and wax out and fresh air in, on the worst of the ears. I've never tried this operation before but I'd like to have a go, especially as the BBC will be here next week. The only real problem is cost, because even if we try to keep it down to a minimum, it'll still be about £150, which she can't afford. I've told her I'll talk to Ian about it and see if she can pay weekly, because Hobo can't go on without having the op done.

Peter from Bullock engineering rang up just now and said that the grassboard axles are ready, so I'll go and pick them up this afternoon and see how they work. I really hope they're OK because I can't afford too many prototypes.

5.00 p.m. I did afternoon surgery, and then there weren't any calls so I went over to pick up the axles. Ian and Keith are really good about letting me go and do things when we're quiet, as long as I've got the mobile phone so if any emergencies come in I'm contactable.

The axles looked pretty good, with the springs fixed in to give some resistance when you lean the board. I bolted them on to the board and headed off to a nearby field to try it out. It's really hard to find suitable hills which aren't private or full of horses or cows. I'm also very conscious of the fact that I'm supposed to be a well-respected member of the local community and shouldn't really be messing around on a piece of plastic on wheels in farmers' fields. I haven't been caught yet, but I can just imagine what some of the local farmers would say if they saw me grassboarding down their prime pasture. I'm not sure they would take my advice on the health of their cattle very seriously after that.

Anyway, I went to a small hill near the practice, with no livestock or farm houses nearby, and had a few runs. It works pretty well, but not quite perfectly yet, I was still overbalancing a lot and it's hard to steer very well. I've got a few ideas about how to improve it, so I'll go back to Peter tomorrow if I get a chance.

Saturday 8 February

1.00 p.m. Hectic morning surgery again. Saturday mornings tend to be really busy at the moment. I think it's because people are off work so they have the time to come down, rather than there is a sudden increase in the number of ill animals every Saturday. I saw a lame golden retriever which is only about eight months old. I think it could be a condition called OCD (or Osteochondritis dissecans to give it its full title), which affects the shoulder, as it occurs in growing, large-breed dogs. It's a disease which attacks the growing cartilage in the joints and can be pretty serious if left untreated. I've told the owners to rest him completely and I've put him on some anti-inflammatory tablets. If he hasn't improved by next week I think I'll have him in to X-ray the joint and see if I can see any cartilage damage, which would confirm the diagnosis. I wonder if Ian would let me operate on it if it needs surgery?

Last night I went over to Dulverton to see Emma. She's just started the lambing season at her practice and work is getting really busy. They tend to do a lot more lambing over there because Exmoor is more suited to sheep farming. She's on call this weekend and she's not looking forward to it. Apparently on busy lambing weekends the vets there don't stop from 7.00 in the morning to 11.00 at night, and then get called out in the middle of the night if they're unlucky. I'm going to head over and see her tonight and take the dogs out tomorrow because she'll probably be too busy to want them around.

Sunday 9 February

9.00 p.m. Emma's had a nightmare of a weekend. When I arrived yesterday afternoon she was out at a lambing, and then she had to go straight off to another one as soon as she got in. That turned out to be a caesar, so it took quite a while. She was pretty pleased with it though because she'd only done one sheep caesar before, and that was with Martin, one of the partners, so this was her first solo one.

Emma's practice is really old fashioned, instead of giving her a mobile phone, she just has an answerphone, so when she's out on a call farmers can only leave messages, they can't actually get through to her. This means that when she gets back from a long visit she can have three or four calls waiting for her to go on, and farmers can wait for hours without even knowing when she'll arrive. I think it's a bad system really, especially for the small-animal clients. It would be dreadful if someone's dog was knocked over or something and they had to wait for hours just to talk to the vet. I suppose things like that are pretty rare, and mobiles don't work too well around Exmoor. It can also be a real pain if someone rings you on the mobile while you're in the middle of calving a cow or something. I had one case a few weeks ago when I was doing a calving for a farmer out near Hartland and a lady rang up to ask me about her budgie. I felt very awkward trying to be nice and helpful to this budgie lady while the big gruff farmer was looking on, waiting for me to get back to his cow.

Today, Emma was out pretty much all day doing lambings, with a few sick calves and one calving thrown in for variety. I took the dogs up on Exmoor for a walk and then headed back here after lunch. I went for a surf, which was excellent because I haven't been in for a while. The surf was quite big but messy and windy, so it wasn't wonderful. It was lovely to come back to a hot shower rather than get out of the sea and have to spend two hours driving back to Bristol.

The BBC are coming tomorrow, which should be good. I hope we can sort out Hobo to operate on while they're here because it'll be an interesting op for them to film. I'd better get my notes out and read up on it so I know what I'm doing. I don't want them to film me making a real mess of it, and I don't want to fail Hobo and Mrs Hartley.

Monday 10 February

8.30 a.m. BBC have arrived to take some shots of me leaving the house. They've set up a camera on a tripod in the car park and are waiting for me to leave and drive off to work.

8.35 a.m. Back again. Apparently I drove off too fast and they didn't get a good enough shot, so they asked me to repeat it.

8.38 a.m. Now they want it from a different angle! I thought this was supposed to be 'fly on the wall', not a scripted drama series.

11.00 a.m. I finally made it to work at about five to nine after they made me stop and do some 'drive by' shots on the way in. I've just nipped home to pick up my surgery textbook so I can check what I'm doing with Hobo.

1.30 p.m. Home for lunch. Hobo's op went really well. He was on his best TV behaviour again, and didn't bite anyone as we gave him his anaesthetic. Once he was asleep I had a careful look at his ear and checked with the book to see exactly what I had to do. It looked straightforward enough in the book, but once he was covered in sterile drapes and I had to decide exactly where to make the first cut, I realized it was going to be more difficult and stressful than I had anticipated.

The camera crew were all crammed into the operating theatre as well, which didn't help matters, and Sarah the director was asking lots of questions while I operated which I found hard to answer and concentrate on the op at the same time. Despite all this, it seemed to go pretty well, all the edges came together OK and the result looked quite respectable. Ian came in at the end and said he thought it was fine. He doesn't seem to mind the cameras too much and ended up chatting away to Sarah about how it was when he first qualified.

Although the op went fine, there could still be complications such as infection and wound breakdown, or it may just not be effective, so it's going to be a difficult few weeks waiting to see how it turns out. I just hope, for my, Hobo's and Mrs Hartley's sakes, that it does work out OK.

6.30 p.m. Hobo went home this evening. We tied his ears together over the top of his head with some sticky bandage so that the wound was open to the fresh air, and his ear wasn't rubbing on it. He didn't think too much of this and had a little nip at Jamie (one of the nurses) when she fetched him from his kennel. Mrs Hartley was also a bit surprised when she saw him, but I explained why he was like that and asked her to bring him back for a check-up in a couple of days, by which time we'll probably be able to let him have his ears down again.

Emma's coming over and the BBC are taking us out for a meal, which should be good. I think they owe me something after all this morning's messing around.

Wednesday 12 February

Nothing much exciting happened yesterday. The BBC followed me to a few farms and filmed a few consultations but I don't think any of the cases were interesting enough to follow up. They went off and filmed Hobo and Mrs Hartley at home, and did some GVs (general views) of Bideford.

*

This morning, Hobo came in for his check-up and was looking excellent, although he had got his ears down within minutes of getting home on Monday. The wound is fine, and he even let me clean it a little without savaging me, which is a good sign. Mrs Hartley was very happy with his progress. The BBC interviewed her in the waiting room, and she was talking about Hobo and the op and how much he meant to her and things. I told her it was looking fine but that the real proof of success wouldn't come for a few more weeks until it was all healed up and the ear was clean and not painful.

They filmed a few other interesting cases today, including a very sick pig and a hen with a scabby foot. The hen was quite good because it decided that it didn't want to be examined and jumped off the consulting table and headed off for a tour of the practice. When I finally caught it, it thanked me by messing all down my trousers, which I didn't think was amusing but everyone else did. I suppose it'll make good television viewing!

They want to set up a romantic meal for Emma and me on Valentine's Day so they can film us together. We're very happy with that, because it means that we get a free meal in a lovely restaurant!

On call tonight. The BBC are itching for a late-night cow caesar or something, but I'm hoping for a nice quiet night in front of the telly.

Thursday 13 February

8.00 a.m. Only one call last night, and that was just someone worrying because their dog was limping slightly. I told them to bring him up today if he's still bad, but I bet he's fine now and they don't bother.

1.00 p.m. Hobo came back in this morning because Mrs Hartley was worried that he was in a lot of pain. She said he was crying and not eating very well. I checked him over and he seems OK, although the ear is pretty tender. His temperature is normal, which is a relief because if it had been up it could have suggested that infection was taking hold. I gave him a painkilling injection and gave her a supply of tablets for him.

7.00 p.m. I took the grassboard back to Peter Bullock this afternoon and explained the problems I was having with the prototype. I told the BBC about the grassboard and they seemed interested in following the story, so they came and filmed me and Peter chatting about it. I hope they continue to film me developing the idea because it'll be great publicity if it gets shown on national telly.

Peter seems to think that we can overcome the problem fairly easily, so he's going to have a go and give me a ring when he's sorted it out. Sarah said that once it's fully working, they'll come and film me riding it. I'm going to look like such a mad eccentric on this programme!

Friday 14 February

8.40 a.m. One Valentine's card, from Emma I think. No surprise flood of cards from grateful female owners though. Never mind, there's always next year.

12.50 a.m. Excellent morning. A lady brought Jerry, a budgie with a broken toe, into morning surgery and the BBC immediately came and filmed the consultation. They seem to love anything involving animals which they perceive to be exotic or interesting. The budgie's toe was beyond repair so I said to the owner that we would anaesthetize him and remove it. I told her that the anaesthetic was the main risk, rather than the op, but we didn't really have a choice, we couldn't remove it with the bird awake.

This was the first bird I've ever anaesthetized on my own. I'd seen it done as a student seeing practice, and thought it didn't look too difficult. What I'd seen other vets use was a special chamber which could be filled with gas, which knocks out the bird without having to use a mask, which can be very stressful for it and very unpleasant for the vet as gas escapes all around the mask and can start to anaesthetize anyone standing nearby. We haven't got one of these chambers, so I decided to improvise using an old ice-cream tub and some sticky tape. I cut a hole in the lid so the gas pipe could be fixed in place with some tape, and another in one side to put the scavenger pipe to take away the old gas. I had some little doubts about the BBC filming the whole affair: my reputation as an eccentric would not be improved by the nation seeing me trying to knock out a bird in a bodged-up anaesthetic box made from an old ice-cream tub.

When the chamber was ready I fetched Jerry and put him in the tub and shut the lid. Jamie turned on the gas and we waited. I confidently expected to hear a nice 'thud' in a few seconds when he fell asleep. After five minutes with no obvious movement I peeked into the box and saw that, far from lying peacefully on the bottom of the tub, he was standing alert, ready to fly off at any moment. We turned up the gas concentration and waited again. After another few minutes I lifted the lid to see Jerry lying down, apparently fast asleep. However, when I reached in to pick him up, he suddenly flapped his wings and flew straight out of the box and started lapping the operating theatre. The camera crew were capturing every moment as what should have been a professional operation descended into a chaotic farce!

Jerry finally settled in one corner of the room and I managed to recapture him by throwing a towel over him before he could launch off again.

This time we took no chances and turned the gas right up, and left him in the box until he was definitely asleep. Then I took him out and very quickly removed the broken toe. The actual operation took about two minutes whereas administering the anaesthetic had taken about an hour!

He recovered well and should be OK. I didn't feel too

bad about the whole mess because, in the end, Jerry was fine and the op had worked. It was pretty badly handled by me, but it was also quite funny and should make a good story for the BBC. If Jerry had died or something then I would have felt bad about doing the whole thing so lightheartedly, but it worked out all right and, even though I'll probably come across as an incompetent madman, at least I won't be an incompetent budgie-murdering madman!

7.00 p.m. Emma's just arrived and we're getting ready to go out for our romantic BBC-organized dinner. We're both quite nervous about being filmed in a pub, it could turn out to be really embarrassing.

Saturday 15 February

8.40 a.m. I am not feeling at my best this morning. Last night was excellent. We went to a really nice pub for the meal and drank too much, all at the BBC's expense! In return they got to film us while we ate, but that wasn't too bad. We felt pretty self-conscious to begin with when they all trooped in and set up cameras and tripods and stuff, and when Sarah was interviewing us, but once we got used to it, it was OK.

The BBC have gone this morning. They seemed pretty pleased with what they filmed and are going to film with Emma in the next couple of weeks. I'm on call all weekend, which I'm not looking forward to at all. The surf's looking good and I'm going to be stuck in the house waiting for the phone to ring.

8.15 p.m. So far so good, only one visit so far and that was just to see a couple of calves with pneumonia.

Being on call is such a pain, even if you're not actually being called out. You can't relax at all, or get stuck into anything, because at any minute the phone *could* ring and you'll have to rush off somewhere. I think it's the worst part of being a vet: it ruins your social life and really limits what you can do outside your job.

Monday 17 February

The weekend was really quiet, which was a relief. Emma came over on Sunday and we took the dogs for a long walk up on the headland. The only call I had on Sunday was to see a vomiting dog in Northam, which wasn't too bad, and that was at 6 p.m. so I didn't mind too much.

Today was pretty busy, I spent most of the morning doing routine farm work and then did afternoon surgery, which was packed. Tonight I'm driving over to Dulverton to play in a pool match with Emma. We've started playing in the local pub team and we're up against the league leaders from Bampton this evening. Our team is pretty poor, and I think we're bottom of our league at the moment, but it's really good fun.

Tuesday 18 February

7.30 a.m. Dulverton We lost horribly last night. I needed to pot a black to win my game but I couldn't hold my nerve in the high-pressure situation and missed it. Emma won hers, but everyone else lost. Our barman has caused a huge row by reporting Bampton to the league for having an under-age player in their team. Everyone, including our team, thinks that he's going too far by reporting them. After all, if the boy's good enough to be playing, then where's the problem? (And he was good enough, he won all of his games easily.) We've got to play them again next week, but away this time. I'm not looking forward to going to their pub after all the bad feeling that's been created. We'll get lynched!

10.30 p.m. I had to go on a house visit out at Hartland this afternoon. I drove out there in some of the worst weather

I've seen since I've been here. The wind was blowing a gale and the rain was pouring down, making it really hard to drive and soaking me when I got out of the car. The wind was so strong that I really had to struggle to get across the car park to Mr and Mrs Gemmill's house, where I was going to see their Westie called Laddie.

The Gemmills turned out to be a lovely couple in their seventies. Laddie had been suffering from collapsing fits over the last few weeks, and apparently they were getting worse. Today, they told me, he was so weak that he had hardly moved for much of the day.

I examined him and couldn't find too much wrong: his heart sounded fine, which made any form of heart failure less likely; his temperature was normal, ruling out infections; and there were no obvious clinical signs to give any clue as to the cause of his weakness. I decided to take some blood and check to see if he had any internal metabolic problems which could cause these symptoms.

I had to ask Mrs Gemmill to raise his vein by pressing in the angle of his elbow, which she didn't seem to mind, and after a few attempts I got a decent blood sample. I gave him a couple of fairly non-specific injections to try and help him over the next few hours and took the blood back to the surgery.

We've got a machine there for analysing blood samples which is excellent, because at a lot of places you still have to send the samples off to a lab and you don't get the results for a couple of days. I ran Laddie's blood through the machine and got the results within about twenty minutes.

They showed that the reason for his collapsing fits was that his blood glucose was really low. This is pretty rare and is most common in animals or humans that are diabetic and overdose on insulin. Laddie wasn't taking insulin so, after looking through a textbook, I decided that the only other possibility was an insulin-producing tumour called an insulinoma. This would cause him to have a low blood glucose level, which in turn causes weakness and collapse. I was very excited by these results as it's not that often that blood results really show such a clear diagnosis. Usually you get a vague idea of what the problem is, or it rules out a few possibilities, but rarely do you actually come up with such an immediate answer.

I rang Mrs Gemmill and told her what I'd found. She was quite upset when I mentioned the word 'tumour', but I explained that it was unlikely to spread or cause any other problems and we should be able to control his symptoms by simply giving him extra sugar. I told her to add some glucose to his water and to put some honey on his tongue whenever he had one of his collapsing episodes

This should sort him out, although he is pretty old so he may not pull through. I hope he does, though, because they're lovely people and I can see that they'd really miss him if he died.

Wednesday 19 February

Terrible news! Ian and Keith have booked me in for a course at the Ministry of Agriculture, Fisheries and Food centre in Exeter next week to learn how to be an LVI (Local Veterinary Inspector). Not only will the course be a day of sheer boredom by all accounts, but being an LVI means that I can do TB testing, which is arguably the dullest job in large-animal vet work. TB testing involves spending one day measuring the skin thickness of all the cows in a herd, then injecting them with bovine and avian TB, followed three days later by measuring them all again to see if there has been any reaction to the injections. It can take anything from a couple of hours to an entire day to get through a herd, depending on the size of the herd and the quality of the handling facilities.

You're not allowed to become an LVI until six months after you qualify, so Ian and Keith have been doing all the testing through the winter. I thought they had forgotten about me and I might get away with not doing any, but Ian dropped the bombshell this morning that I was all booked up and expected in Exeter at 9.00 a.m. next Thursday.

I rang Emma because she's already done the course and has done a few tests. She said the course was very boring, but that there were up sides to being an LVI, such as the power to order any animal carcass to be exhumed, the ability to order the seizure of any meat products and being able to set off a national panic by diagnosing foot and mouth disease in a herd of cattle! I like the idea of being able to order the seizure of any meat products – when I'm an LVI I'm going to go to Tesco's and seize all their prime steak!

Thursday 20 February

8.30 a.m. On call again last night. I had to go out and see a horse which had got a piece of carrot stuck in its throat. We don't see many horses at this practice so I always feel quite nervous when I have to go and see them. I think it's because I wasn't brought up with horses so I don't know all the horsey terms and I can't really relate to horse owners as well as I do to farmers.

I suppose it's really only because I've had a lot to do with farmers and I feel quite confident about knowing what I'm talking about where farm matters are concerned. With horses, I always have a sneaking suspicion that the owners know more then I do and that I'll make a terrible mistake and either kill the horse, or look stupid in front of the owner. It must be the same for vets who see lots of horses but don't go to many farms: they would feel just as uneasy treating cows and dealing with the farmers.

When I arrived at the house they took me up a dark winding path to the paddock where the horse was kept.

'He's a bit wild; we don't handle him very much,' warned Mrs Weeks, the mother of the large family of excited children who had gathered around to see the vet in action.

'He bites!' added one of the kids.

One of the eldest children volunteered to catch Rascal the pony, and proceeded to spend the next twenty minutes chasing him around the paddock in the dark. Eventually the pony was caught and I examined him. With a fading torch beam I could just see a piece of carrot wedged in Rascal's throat. I grabbed his tongue and pulled it out of his mouth to keep him from biting, and very quickly reached in and extracted the carrot.

Relieved to have solved the problem without losing any fingers, I headed back to the car feeling quite pleased with myself. The Weeks clan were happy that lovely Rascal was OK, and I was pleased that I wouldn't have to go near him again.

6.15 p.m. Boring day today, lots of routine farm calls and a few pretty dull consultations. Emma from the BBC rang to see if they could come back in a couple of weeks, which I said should be fine. Hopefully the grassboard will be up and running by then so they can film me cruising majestically down some hills. Well, bouncing down on my backside with bits of grassboard all around is probably more likely!

Friday 21 February

Mrs Hartley brought Hobo in this morning to have his stitches out. The wound is looking excellent, and the ear is much cleaner and less sore than before the op. He wasn't too keen on having the stitches taken out because there were about twenty in total, most of which were right down in his ear canal and pretty painful to remove.

After Mrs Hartley left, Sue, the receptionist, came in and said that she had left me a little present to say thank you for what we'd done for Hobo. I unwrapped the package to find a lovely home-made paperweight. It's a base with some model animals and plants fixed on top to create a country scene. I'm not sure exactly what to do with it, but it's a lovely thought, and she's obviously put loads of time and effort into it. It's really nice when clients appreciate what you do for them, rather than moan and whinge about cost all the time.

Before I qualified I had this romantic picture of being a country vet where all the clients gave you bottles of whisky and wine, and all the farmers paid you in kind with a side of beef or a couple of large cheeses. I found out pretty quickly that this isn't the case nowadays. Although you do get the odd bottle of wine or box of chocolates, most small-animal clients seem to be much more business-like. I think it's a reflection of how things have changed since the days of James Herriot, not just in terms of how clients treat the vet, but a general change in attitude from the vet being an important social figure who looked after the community's animals, to the vet who is part of a small business, competing in a modern market-place. People see their vet now as a necessary service to be paid for in much the same way as a garage is essential for maintaining cars. This is good in many ways: it means that vets are more accountable and have to offer a decent service to keep clients, but it is sad, none the less, that the magic and mystique have largely gone from the profession.

Emma and I are off to Kent to spend the weekend at her home. Her family are lovely, I get on really well with them, so it's not like going to spend a terrible few days with the dreaded in-laws or anything. It'll be good to get away from Devon for a while as well because, although I love it here, it's nice to get a change of scenery every now and then.

Monday 24 February

1.20 p.m. We had a brilliant weekend. Too much to drink and we spent too much money, but so good to get away and see some other people rather than just other vets and clients.

It was terrible going back to work this morning after

such a good few days off, especially as morning surgery was packed. Then, to cap it all, I had to go out to Brian Hill at Hartland and see three horribly lame cows. It was the same old story: problems which had been left too long and had gone beyond the stage where they were really treatable. One of them was so bad in both back feet that I had to recommend it was slaughtered because it was in so much pain. It really is disgusting that these animals are allowed to get into this state; if we'd seen them a few weeks back, we probably could have saved them. This farmer has got the attitude that the vet is too expensive, and why bother unless it's really essential? Which is silly and unfair on the animals he's supposed to be looking after.

After struggling around in the mud at Mr Hill's for an hour or so, I popped in to see Mr and Mrs Gemmill to check on Laddie. They were very pleased to see me and seemed happy with his progress.

'Oh, he's wonderful. He's not having nearly so many of his little fits now, and he's much brighter in himself.' Mr Gemmill beamed.

I stayed for a while and checked him over, and he really did seem much more lively and happier. It felt so good to think I'd helped this dog and by doing so helped its owners. I can't quite believe that such an unusual and rare diagnosis seems to be right and that the simple treatment is working so well.

The Gemmills are such a nice couple, they made me coffee and really treated me with respect. I take back some of what I said a few days ago about the way the client–vet relationship has changed in recent years; this case and others, like Jake Johnson, may be exceptions nowadays, but they still make being a vet so rewarding and restore your faith in why you are doing it.

When I first decided I wanted to be a vet, I was about fourteen, and I pictured it as being very much like James Herriot. I wanted to work out in the beautiful countryside, dealing with friendly farmers and interesting animals. I saw being a vet as more than just a job; it was a way of life which would be both exciting and rewarding. Certainly for me, and probably for a lot of vets in my generation, the main influences behind the desire to become a vet were the James Herriot books and TV programmes. They portrayed such an idyllic picture of life that I'm sure they inspired many children to try and follow in Herriot's footsteps. Now that I am a vet, I suppose I'm sometimes disappointed by the realities of the job. It has changed an awful lot since the days described by James Herriot, and what I do now is very different to what he did back in the thirties and forties. Although it isn't what I dreamt of as a child, it is still a very special profession and I don't think there are any other jobs quite like it. It can get very dull and routine, but then you get a case like Laddie that really reminds you why you wanted to be a vet in the first place.

Tuesday 25 February

I spent most of today doing farm work. One of the calls was to a farmer over near Torrington called Philip Morris. His farm is a well-run medium-size dairy farm, and we do quite a lot of scanning and general routine work there. He's a really friendly farmer, and we normally get chatting about all sorts of stuff while I'm working away on his cows. We started talking about BSE this morning and how it's affected dairy farming round here. He was saying that, although it's meant a drop in the price of beef and milk to some extent, it hasn't affected diary farmers too much. Beef farmers have been much worse off because all of their income comes from selling beef, whereas dairy farmers only get a small part of their income from beef calves and get most of their money from milk sales, which haven't been affected too badly by the crisis.

I suppose it has even had some benefits because since the

new regulations have come in to try and get rid of all animals over thirty months old from the food chain, farmers have been getting really good prices for older cows when normally they would be worth very little. Now, instead of older cows fetching almost nothing for meat, or at the knackers, the government pays a decent amount to encourage the destruction of these older animals. It has changed our work as well to some degree because, before all this happened, farmers would be more inclined to treat cows when they were ill, whereas, now they can get a good price for them on the over-thirty-month scheme, they are tending to have them slaughtered and take the money rather than try to treat them. This means that we are signing many more slaughter certificates and treating fewer animals, which is pretty frustrating and unrewarding but is good in some respects because farmers with lots of very lame or old and decrepit animals can afford to replace them with younger, healthier animals rather than keep them going when they really should be slaughtered.

I stayed at Philip's farm for as long as possible to try and avoid doing a visit to an awkward old man in Bideford (perfectly healthy cairn terrier, which bites, and an owner who is convinced that the dog is suffering from all sorts of obscure diseases), which had been booked in this morning. I should have guessed that it would still be waiting for me when I got back so I ended up having hardly any lunch break as a result. I suppose it's because I'm the assistant and Keith and Ian are the partners, but I get a bit annoyed by the way the work is shared out sometimes. I always seem to be first in line to do any calls, and only if I'm busy will they go out. If I was the boss I'd probably do the same, though, thinking about it; there's no point having a dog and barking yourself, as my boss in Australia used to say when he was getting me to do the worst jobs on the farm.

Wednesday 26 February

4.30 p.m. On call this evening, so I've got to do surgery in half an hour's time. I've just spent most of the afternoon trying to clean the inside of my car. It's been getting more and more smelly over the past few weeks and I think I've found out why. The back seat, where the dogs sit, has got soaked in wet dog juice, and when I took it out, the foam of the seat has gone mouldy and absolutely stinks. I've taken the whole thing out and put it next to a heater to dry, but I have a feeling that the damage is done and it may never recover. The boot was in a pretty horrible state as well, everything is a real mess and it smells like an abattoir! I think what I may do is build an organizer box for the boot so that I can get everything sorted out and try to keep it reasonably clean and smell free.

11.00 p.m. One call out to see an itchy cat in Westward Ho!, but quiet apart from that. I spent the rest of the evening designing my new boot-organizer box. If my first prototype is a success, maybe I can market the idea. The Inglis Vet Box, yours for a mere £299.99 plus P&P, guaranteed to keep your boot organized and clean!

11.15 p.m. Oh no! I've just remembered what I'm doing tomorrow, the bloody LVI course in Exeter.

Thursday 27 February

8.00 p.m. Just got home from the LVI day, which was as bad as expected. The only good part was meeting some of the other new vets who were on the course as well. A couple were in my year at Bristol, so it was good to see them again.

The morning was spent at the centre in Exeter learning about the theory behind TB testing, filling out import and export forms, and notifiable diseases. In the afternoon we drove out to the field station to look at some slides and be given a guided tour of the place and shown how they deal with all the samples that we vets send in to them.

I suppose it was quite useful, but most of it was very dull and boring. It seems to be 95 per cent paperwork and only a little bit of useful, interesting vet work, but I suppose it's all necessary and what seem to be dull, repetitive, pointless procedures have in fact been the reason why TB is under control (well, nearly under control) and why the UK is free from most really nasty animal diseases that cause loads of problems elsewhere in the world.

I am now a fully qualified Local Veterinary Inspector, and I have a list of powers ranging from declaring a farm an infected area and closing down all animal movement within ten miles, to organizing the export of dogs to far-off countries. I am a government employee! In reality I think the limit of my new high-powered duties will be doing TB and other tests, but you never know. I could be out at a farm one day and see a case of foot and mouth disease, in which case I'd have to shut the farm, call the police and the ministry and stand guard until they arrived. It's quite unlikely, seeing that the last recorded case was in the sixties.

Friday 28 February

I used my new powers for the first time today. Mr Palmer, a farmer from Alvediscott, had a cow which had died suddenly overnight and I had to go and take a blood sample to check for anthrax. I brought the blood back to the surgery and made a smear on a slide and stained it to show up any bacteria. Under the microscope I could see lots of normal bacteria, but none of the tell-tale chains of encapsulated rods which would indicate anthrax. I was a bit disappointed really; after all the long talks yesterday about what to do in the event of diagnosing anthrax, how to dispose of the carcass safely, and all the other associated procedures, it was a little dull just to fill in the form saying 'negative'. The brief excitement of doing my first ministry work soon wore off as I had to fill in a pile of forms to record the test and claim for the mileage and fees for doing it (not that I see any of the money, it goes straight into the practice coffers).

Ian has booked my first TB test for the week after next. I have to do my first one under the supervision of a ministry vet, to make sure I get it right. Quite how hard it can be to measure the skin and do a couple of injections I don't know, but I suppose it's pretty vital to be accurate. If you make a mistake, it could lead to the farmer having movement restrictions placed on his farm until a re-test is done, which would be very bad news for him.

March

Saturday 1 March

12.30 p.m. Just finished morning surgery, so I'm off until Monday now. My dad is coming down this afternoon for the weekend, which should be good. He's only been down once before and that was in September last year so it'll be great to see him again.

The surf is looking promising so I think I'll have to persuade Dad to look after the dogs for an hour or two while I have a quick surf.

4.00 p.m. Dad was late, as usual, so I didn't feel too guilty about roping him in to walking Pan and Badger on the beach while I had a surf. He's not really a dog lover but he seems to get on with our two pretty well. They're so obedient, even with people they don't know, which makes walking them so much more fun for them and whoever is doing the walking.

It really annoys me to see all the dogs being walked on the beach and Northam Burrows pulling away at their leads because their owners can't control them if they let them off. How much fun can it be for the dog to be taken for a walk where they can't even run about and exercise? Dogs really enjoy trotting off and having a good sniff and an explore, and I think it's cruel to deny them this pleasure, especially when so many dogs are left alone for most of the day anyway. If owners just followed a few basic rules of training when they are bringing up their dogs, such as ensuring that the dog knows that you are the boss and leader of the pack, then everyone could have a well-adjusted, obedient pet, rather than a messed-up animal who refuses to come when called and is generally disobedient and unhappy as a result.

I think the biggest mistake people make is treating their dog too much like an equal and not as a lower member of the group. Dogs are naturally pack animals and in the wild organize themselves into a pack with a definite hierarchy, so each animal knows where it stands in the order and who to obey. Domestic dogs as pets need to know that they are bottom of the family pack, otherwise they tend to become disobedient. Being bottom dog doesn't mean being unhappy. Far from it. If they know their place, they can be happy and content without the stresses and strains of trying to assert dominance.

Far too many owners fail to show their dog their authority and end up with a dog who may become aggressive because it doesn't respect its owner as 'top dog'. Showing dominance doesn't mean hitting the dog or anything like that, it just means making sure it always obeys your orders and does what it's told. After a short time this will become ingrained and the dog will be naturally obedient and content as a result.

I must stop rambling on and on about things like this. It does annoy me, though, maybe I should do something positive about it and write a book on dog training and the general evils of the average dog owner. Maybe not, I could lose all my clients pretty quickly!

Sunday 2 March

6.00 p.m. Emma came over last night and we all went out for an excellent pub meal in Buckland Brewer, a small village a couple of miles away.

Today we went for a walk out at Hartland Quay, which was really nice. The dogs love it there, lots of interesting smells and horse dung to roll in (my car is starting to smell again). I spotted some great-looking grassboarding hills. I can't wait to come and try it out on some places like this. There's so much potential for people to take their boards and head off and find a hill somewhere and have fun. Snowboarding is fantastic, but you have to travel all the way to Europe or the States to do it, and it costs a fortune. You can go on the dry skiing slopes, but they're lethal. The only time I've tried boarding on a dry slope I broke my thumb. It was then I decided that it must be possible to create a snowboard for grass, after all, grass is much softer than dry slope material, and it's everywhere.

I hope that the grassboard works out and I can really make something which acts like snowboarding on grass. It's not that I want to get rich really (although that would be rather nice if it happened), I just want to be proved right, and see people riding the hills everywhere on my invention in a few years' time.

Dad is staying this evening because he's got tomorrow off work, so we're going to have a meal in and then head up to the local for a couple of pints later on.

Monday 3 March

7.55 a.m. Oh, my head!

8.00 a.m. Why did Dad force me to stay at the pub for that extra pint?

8.15 a.m. It's no good, I'm going to have to get up and face Monday morning. It's all right for Dad, he can stay in bed all morning and then drive gently home. I've got a morning surgery, which is bound to be busy, followed by a massive load of castrating and disbudding at Hescott's farm.

1.00 p.m. I survived the morning! I think a couple of hours' hard physical work outside was just what I needed to get rid of the hangover, although the first couple of castrations were a little unpleasant. I like Mr Hescott, which always makes things better. He was telling me about his farm dogs, which are all lovely collies, and how useful they are around the farm. They never disappear off or cause trouble and are really obedient, especially when they're working. They also look so much more contented than most pet dogs. I think that's because they know their place and have a feeling of working within a pack. If I was a dog I'd much rather be one of Mr Hescott's farm collies and put up with cheap dog food, hard work and a cold bed, than be a pampered pooch living on choice steak, sleeping in a luxury bed but having little exercise or fun.

9.00 p.m. Not such a bad day after all. This afternoon I went back to pick up MkIII grassboard, which is looking much better thanks to the modifications Peter has made. I tried it out in a small park in Bideford which I spotted yesterday. The board and the new hill were both excellent. The board now turns much better and I wasn't falling over nearly as much, and the hill is perfect – just the right amount of slope and nice short, even grass. I'll have to take it to the hill Dad and I spotted on Sunday at Hartland Quay next time I'm on a call out that way.

Tuesday 4 March

12.30 p.m. I had some really bad news this morning. Laddie, Mr and Mrs Gemmill's dog, died overnight. Apparently he had been doing really well and hardly collapsing at all, so they were really shocked and upset when they found him this morning. I was out near Hartland anyway so I popped in to see them after finishing my calls.

They were so nice and understanding, and didn't try to blame me for what had happened. They kept thanking me for what I'd done and saying that he'd had a good couple of weeks thanks to the tests we'd done, but I still felt as if I'd let them down. Maybe I'd misinterpreted the blood results, or maybe there was some other treatment which I'd not used which could have helped. It always seems to be the nicest clients whose animals get the worst illnesses or don't respond to treatment as they should, and the clients who are hard to deal with and unfriendly have all the luck.

I'm getting a bit more used to dealing with animals dying,

but it's still upsetting and makes you question your own abilities. Once I get more self-confidence in my skills of diagnosing and treating animals, hopefully I will be able to tell myself that I'd done everything possible and actually believe it, without the nagging self-doubt which seems to be there at the moment.

7.00 p.m. Cheered up a bit this afternoon. I did my first lambing as a qualified vet; good to have under my belt.

The farmer, Mr Ashford, brought in one of his pedigree Suffolk ewes, which had been trying to lamb since this morning. Mr Ashford only has eighteen ewes, as he is a retired teacher, I think, and just indulges in a bit of farming as a hobby. He isn't a very experienced farmer, so he'd only had a quick feel inside and then brought her down to us. As it turned out, it was a very simple case of one leg being in the wrong place, and it only took a couple of minutes to sort it out and pull out the lamb. There was another live lamb behind the first so Mr Ashford was very happy with the result, and I was pleased to have had such an easy lambing for my first one.

Wednesday 5 March

1.00 p.m. Morning surgery was pretty busy today, this is what I saw:

> cat with mild cat flu, antibiotics, see again in four days
> two cats for boosters
> dog lame in right hind leg, nothing obvious so given anti-inflammatory and antibiotic injections – should be fine
> dog with skin rash, antibiotics and prednisolone tablets, see again next week
> cat been in fight, admit to lance abscess on face
> dog booster plus kennel cough (little terrier, bit nurse as we were squirting the vaccine up its nose)

clip rabbit's teeth
dog with conjunctivitis, antibiotic eye ointment,
   check in two days

After morning surgery I did a couple of ops: a bitch spay and a dog castration. The bitch spay was a big golden retriever and it was the most difficult one I've done yet because everything was very fat inside and the ovarian stumps kept tearing and oozing. The hardest bit of a bitch spay is getting the ligatures around the ovarian stumps because they are so awkward to get access to, and if the dog is fat, it makes things even harder. I was pretty worried until she woke up, but she seems fine now, and her colour looks good, so hopefully there's no internal bleeding.

4.30 p.m. Bonnie (the bitch spay) has just been picked up by her owner and I'm very relieved that she's OK.

Nothing much else happened this afternoon, except for a visit by a drugs rep, who gave us all free towels and pens. The towels will come in very handy for trying to protect what remains of the back seat of the car.

7.00 p.m. I have had an absolute nightmare of an evening. I was just about to leave at 5 p.m. when Mrs Lawrence rushed back into the car park and carried Bonnie into the surgery with blood literally pouring out of the wound. At first I thought that something else must have happened to her, like being hit by a car or something, but Mrs Lawrence said that on the way home in the car she'd suddenly noticed a pool of blood appear underneath Bonnie as she shifted position on the back seat. She was being remarkably calm (a lot calmer than I was feeling anyway), and listened as I very rapidly explained that we'd have to get her on a drip and then re-operate to find the bleeding vessel and clamp it off.

Helen, one of the nurses, came and helped me carry her through to the theatre, where we put an i/v line in and started some fluids going in, in an attempt to maintain Bonnie's blood volume. My main worry was that she'd lose too much blood and go into shock. If that happened our chances of saving her would be very slim.

As soon as we had the fluids going, I gave her as small a dose of anaesthetic as I could to get her under and then stabilized her on gas. While I scrubbed up, Helen cleaned as much of the blood away from the wound site as possible and prepped the area ready for me to re-enter the abdomen.

The abdomen was awash with blood, so it took a long time and a lot of swabs to clear the area sufficiently for me to try and locate the bleeding ovarian vessels. Even with most of the blood gone, it took about quarter of an hour to find and re-ligature each stump, both of which were oozing blood. Only once I'd checked and rechecked each side about half a dozen times was I confident enough to close the wound again.

Helen, meantime, was struggling to keep Bonnie asleep without letting her go too deep and risk not coming round. It's at times like these that you really appreciate good nurses like Helen. If you have confidence in the nurse you can let them get on with the anaesthetic while you concentrate on the operation without having to keep checking on the animal.

She came round from the anaesthetic OK, and by the time I left a few minutes ago, she was sitting up and looking remarkably bright, considering what she'd been through.

I think this has been the most stressful couple of hours of my veterinary career so far, not only because we were battling to save a dog which was really close to not making it, but mainly because it was entirely my fault. I know that most vets have a few bleeding bitch spays when they first start, and even experienced vets have the occasional problem, but that doesn't make me feel any better. Bonnie's a lovely dog, with a really nice owner, and if she dies because of my surgery, I'm going to feel so dreadful and so guilty.

11.30 p.m. Just been in to check on Bonnie and she's looking fine. I spoke to Mrs Lawrence on the phone earlier and explained what had happened and how she was recovering. She was still very calm and understanding, which is surprising considering what has happened to her dog.

Thursday 6 March

8.30 a.m. I've just been up to the surgery and Bonnie's OK! I don't think I've ever been so relieved in all my life. She's sitting up, looking bright and alert as if to say, 'What was all the fuss about? Of course I'm OK.' I felt very grateful to her for pulling through, a lesser dog may well have not survived such a large amount of blood loss and a second big operation.

I rang Mrs Lawrence and she was very happy. She's coming down to pick her up later on this morning. We're not going to charge her for what we did, because it was due to my mistake. In some cases, where an animal has a complication after an operation which is nobody's fault, we do have to charge for any subsequent treatment, but in cases like this it would be very hard to justify charging the owner.

1.00 p.m. Bonnie went home looking remarkably well. Mrs Lawrence was so understanding and didn't blame me at all. She said her brother is a vet and she spoke to him about what had happened, and he told her that it was just one of those things that can happen and Bonnie had simply been unlucky. I'm grateful to him for not turning round and saying, 'That's terrible, you should sue your incompetent vet,' but I still feel I'm to blame. I think I've been incredibly lucky and hopefully I've learnt from this experience and won't let it happen again. Another time I may not be so fortunate, either in the outcome, or in the owner.

Friday 7 March

Last night Emma came over and I told her all about Bonnie and what had happened. She said she'd had a couple of nasty bleeding spays, so it wasn't just me. She also told me she'd heard some horror stories from other people who had qualified with us. One girl, Kate, was working in a really old-fashioned practice somewhere in Wales, and when she'd first started there she'd had a couple of bitch spays die because they'd been bleeding a little bit when she was operating. Apparently she'd asked her boss what to do and instead of telling her to find the bleeding vessel and re-ligature it, he'd just told her to close the animal up and said, 'Oh, she'll be OK.' In the first two cases the animals weren't OK and died in recovery, and since then Kate has decided to ignore her boss's advice and now rigorously checks all her spays for bleeding before closing them up.

It's strange how vets vary in their standards and techniques. There is definitely a spectrum of vets ranging from what I would consider to be really poor to exceptionally good. Often the clients will never know if their vet is a brilliant or a terrible vet, because the only factor they can gauge is how the vet comes across to the client. You can get vets with a fantastic kennel-side manner who are by no means fantastic surgeons and others who really have a problem communicating with their clients and may come across as rude or incompetent, but are in fact superb veterinarians (just like doctors I suppose).

I hope I'm somewhere in the middle, I know my standard of medicine and surgery is not any way near as good as some vets', but I think I can communicate fairly well with clients, and that goes a long way to being a reasonable all-rounder. A large part of being a successful vet in the eyes of your clients is the ability to communicate with them, and your technical skills and medical knowledge are, in a way, secondary to this. I'm not sure this is how it should be, but being a vet is a very public profession, and if you can't talk to your clients then you can't give a good all-round service, even if you can recite the textbooks backwards.

Monday 10 March

8.30 a.m. I was on call over the weekend and it was pretty busy. On Saturday I had a full morning surgery followed by a couple of farm visits, then in the afternoon I had to see a couple of ill dogs and put a cat to sleep. Yesterday I had to do a calving, a milk fever and see a dog with a broken nail.

In general I get things fairly easy when I'm on call compared to some of my friends. Tom, who is working in Exeter, told me that on an average he gets about twenty to twenty-five calls each day if he's on at the weekend, whereas I tend to get maybe three or four if I'm unlucky. I had one weekend soon after I started when the only call I had all weekend was a worried goldfish owner, but that was exceptionally quiet. The worst thing is that however quiet you are the phone could always ring at any time day or night, so you never quite relax until they are handed back to the nurses at 8.15 a.m. on Monday.

10.00 a.m. On my way to my first TB test, out at Brian Lee's farm near Stoney Cross. I've been to this farm once before to see some ill calves and I think it's not too bad and the farmer's friendly enough. The one thing I do remember about it is that the old farmer has got one of the strongest Devonshire accents I've ever heard. He also suffers from some lung problem so, as a result, I couldn't understand a word he said last time I was there. I ended up nodding my head and agreeing with everything because I got too embarrassed to keep asking him to repeat himself. I hope his son is there today because I can just about make out what he's saying.

2.30 p.m. Finally finished! What a chaotic morning. There were only seventy-odd cattle to test, which would normally take about an hour or an hour and a half, but it has just taken us nearly four hours!

The problem was that all the cattle were in little separate groups in different sheds, so instead of running all seventy straight through the crush, we had to wait while Brian and his son fetched each group of seven or eight cattle, and then return them to their shed before getting the next batch. Things were made worse by the assistance of Roy, the world's least obedient cattle dog. He is a big farm collie with a bit of Labrador or something in his make-up, and he spent the entire morning getting in the way, barking at the cattle and generally making the whole job a lot more difficult. The only sentences that I could actually understand Brian say all morning were, 'Roy, get over 'ere!' and, 'Roy, no!', neither of which had any discernable effect on what Roy did.

The ministry vet who was there to observe my test and check that all was well was a nice enough bloke who obviously didn't want to be there at all. He had come over from Barnstaple expecting a nice easy couple of hours, and ended up missing his lunch and generally having his day ruined.

The final straw came quite near the end. We'd done all but the last group of animals, which were the oldest bullocks. As Brian was bringing this final group down from their shed, Roy leapt out at them from behind a bale of straw and launched himself at the heels of the first animal.

'Roy! Roy! Leave 'em!' Brian shouted desperately. 'Heel, heel. Come 'ere, Roy!' But it was too late, the biggest bullock, the one being attacked by Roy, turned and headed over the nearest fence, demolishing it in the process.

He didn't stop at that one fence, he disappeared over another fence, through a hedge and into the distance, with Brian and Roy vainly giving chase. Luckily the rest of the bullocks had fled in the opposite direction and we managed to get them safely into a shed, but there was no chance of catching the fleeing animal, who was by now about three fields away and still going.

Brian and the rest of the men got the Land-Rover and took off in pursuit, leaving me and the ministry man to wait.

They eventually returned, without the missing animal, about forty minutes later. The ministry man was getting more and more agitated by the delay and by the time Brian returned he was far from amused by the whole situation. I, on the other hand, was quite happy to be sitting in the sun on a bale, doing nothing, knowing that I'd never make it back in time for afternoon surgery.

Brian explained that the bullock was in another farmer's field about three miles away, but they'd have to take a trailer up to bring him back once he'd calmed down a bit. At least that's what I think he said, his actual words were, 'Ah, 'ee's up in top feeld, ower by 'aaht ould shed. We'll nebutt gerrim till 'ee's a birit less straapy. Ah'I tik the baax up and fetch the lirrel saad tomorrow.'

We decided to finish off the test and leave the escapee until he was recaptured and I would come back to test him on a separate day. The final few animals were pretty excitable after what had happened but, by locking Roy away in the house, we managed to get through them with no more casualties.

I was very relieved to finish and was happily packing away my things when Brian reminded me that we had to repeat the whole lot on Wednesday to read the test.

'I'll bey seeying thee on Wensdye theen,' he said.

I am not looking forward to it.

Tuesday 11 March

Bonnie came in this morning for a check-up and she's fine. I'm not sure if Mrs Lawrence realizes quite how relieved I am, and how close Bonnie came to not making it. Ten more minutes and she may well not have survived, I reckon, but she did, so I shouldn't keep worrying about it – I'll just double or triple check all my ligatures from now on.

It was really quiet today so I've been constructing my boot organizer. I bought some plywood, glue, nails and a saw and spent most of the afternoon in my spare bedroom building what is surely going to be the finest boot box in the country. It's going to be a large wooden box with lots of little compartments and sliding trays to accommodate all the drugs and equipment that are in a jumble in the back of my car at the moment.

We've got the postponed return pool match against Bampton this evening. It was cancelled for a couple of weeks due to the complaint made by our barman. None of us are looking forward to going to their pub, things could get nasty!

Wednesday 12 March

7.15 a.m. Dulverton Mild hangover. Last night's pool match wasn't too bad, although we did lose 6-nil. No fights or anything, although I'm sure they didn't thaw the sausage rolls properly on purpose.

10.30 a.m. Just finished morning surgery and I'm about to go off and face Brian, Roy and the escaping cow. I saw one interesting case in surgery, a cat which is really lame in one of its hind legs. I've admitted it to X-ray later on. I hope I'll be back in time to do it, but if today is anything like Monday, I've got no chance.

1.15 p.m. The test reading was remarkably incident free, mainly because Roy was chained up in the house and Brian was off at market, so his son Steve was in charge, and I could just about understand him.

It was much easier than the first part of the test because instead of having to inject and measure each animal, it was just a case of running them through the handling facilities and measuring any with obvious lumps. As it happened there weren't any reactors or even any inconclusive results, so I didn't have to serve any movement restriction orders (I was a bit disappointed really, I was looking forward to using my new official powers). Steve was very relieved because they've got a big load of fattened cattle ready for market next week and if there'd been any reactors, they wouldn't have been allowed to move any animals off the farm until it had been cleared, which can take up to six months.

The escapee had been recaptured so I did the first part of the test on him and I'll have to come back in two days to measure the result. Steve was taking no chances: in the last couple of days they had replaced the broken section of fence and parked a large tractor in the way just in case he tries his tricks again. He was pretty quiet this time round, though, I think he'd realized that he had no chance of ever making it to freedom and had given up.

As a child I'd always have this little fantasy that if I was a farm animal, I'd escape and go and live in the wild, roaming free in the open country. However, since then I've come to realize that, except in a few places, there is no open wild country for them to escape to even if they wanted to. All the land is farmed or owned or has buildings on it, so there's nowhere for escapee animals to escape too. I suppose also animals like cows and sheep are herd animals and are happiest in large groups, so they don't really have any incentive to break free and head off on their own.

I managed to get back in time to look at the cat. I gave it a quick anaesthetic and palpated its injured leg. With the cat relaxed, it was easier to feel the bones and soft tissues of the leg, and the diagnosis became clear, she had dislocated her hip. I took an X-ray to confirm this, and to make sure that there were no fractures or other injuries. The X-ray showed the ball of the femur sitting above and forward of the socket in the pelvis, but luckily there were no other obvious injuries.

I asked Ian to come and have a look because I'd never tried to reduce a dislocation like this before. He had a quick feel and then with a swift pull and twist I heard a click and the hip was back in.

'There you go,' he said. 'Nothing to it. Just pull like this, and twist the leg, and it'll pop back in.'

'Is that it?' I asked, thinking that there must surely be more to it than a simple pull and twist.

'It should be. Sometimes they come out again, but if it's not been out too long, it'll probably be fine.' He checked the joint to make sure it was still in place. 'If it does keep coming out, we'll have to operate, but they're normally OK.'

I was very impressed, but I suppose he has been doing the job for thirty-five years, so he's probably seen a few of these in his time. Hopefully next time I'll be able to reduce it myself with similar ease, although I bet he made it look a lot easier than it is.

Thursday 13 March

On last night, but no call-outs. I played Keith at squash but lost, which was annoying. It's the same old thing, playing someone twenty years older, who is less fit and looks easy to beat, and getting thrashed. I would really like to win against Keith, there is something about being beaten by him that really gets to me!

Today I went out to Charles Moore's place for routine scanning and fertility work. He reminded me about the nutrition meeting, which is next week. I think I'll go because although it'll probably be pretty dull, it would be good to learn (or re-learn) some nutrition. It's the kind of subject that farmers often ask about and it'd be nice to actually know what I was talking about when I give them advice.

Friday 14 March

2.00 p.m. Another busy morning surgery, which I ended up doing most of as usual. According to the rota it should have been me and Ian on this morning, but Ian tends to do paperwork or something, and only helps if the waiting room is really bulging at the seams. Most of the cases were pretty routine, including:

> four dogs for boosters
> three cats for boosters
> one dog for a nail trim
> one coughing dog (heart trouble)

However, there was one interesting case, which was a cat with a broken leg. It had been out all night and the owners had noticed it wasn't putting one of its back legs to the ground when it came in this morning. Usually when you get a case with a history like that it turns out to be just a sprain or a cat bite or something fairly dull, but in this case as soon as I felt the affected leg I could immediately feel the grating bone, which suggested that the leg was fractured.

'We'll take him in for an X-ray, and then we'll be able to tell a lot more about the chances of fixing it,' I said.

Mrs Thompson, his elderly owner, was quite upset by the whole thing.

I gave him an anaesthetic and took an X-ray. Ian and Keith were both out on calls so I was hoping that the fracture would be a simple one, and that I would be able to have a go at fixing it myself. The X-ray had to be taken up to the hospital for developing, which means a delay of about quarter of an hour between taking the picture and getting the result, during which the animal has to be kept asleep in case another picture is needed. I'm really going to get on to Ian and Keith about getting some form of developer, even if it's just a manual one in the basement.

Anyway, the X-ray showed exactly what I was hoping for, a nice clean break in the middle of the femur, which looked very straightforward to fix with a pin. I kept the cat under the anaesthetic while I sorted out a suitable pin and had a quick flick through a couple of surgery textbooks to refresh my memory on the technique for this operation. It all looked very easy and simple so I decided to get on with it while I had the cat asleep, rather than subjecting it to another anaesthetic later in the day.

I was expecting the op to take about half an hour, but I was still struggling away with the pin nearly two hours later when Ian returned. Things had started well: I'd found the break and pushed the pin up inside the near piece of the bone and out through the skin above the hip. Then I'd pulled the pin almost all the way through so that the pointed end just protruded from the bone. Next I lined up the other piece of bone and pushed the pin in until it was, hopefully, lying in a nice straight line and the tip of the pin was right up to the end of the bone without actually coming through into the knee joint. I couldn't see much, due to the muscle and other tissue in the way, so I took another X-ray at that point to check the alignment of the two pieces of bone and the pin.

Unfortunately, when the X-ray came back from the hospital, it showed that the pin had not passed in a straight line down the far part of the femur, but had instead headed off to one side. The result would be bone which would heal in a crooked manner, possibly leaving the cat with permanent lameness.

I had to open up the wound again and pull the pin back. Then I had to try and get the bones correctly aligned, before pushing the pin into the lower part again. It took quite a while to get the bones finally nicely lined up, but eventually, just as Ian appeared, I got it right. I took a final X-ray, which thankfully confirmed that the leg was properly set, and woke the cat up.

I was exhausted. It should have been a quick and easy operation, but it had taken nearly two hours and left me feeling drained from the tension. I think, in future, I might wait for some advice and supervision before attempting something new like this. I'm sure Ian could have saved me about an hour by advising me on exactly how to do the operation.

Ian was quite impressed by the end result. I told him I'd only started forty minutes ago so that he didn't think I'd been making a mess of it. Unfortunately he found the X-ray of the first pinning attempt which gave the game away somewhat, but he wasn't annoyed at all, he just said that he was glad it had turned out OK.

I'm off for the weekend now, so I'll have to leave the cat and hope she recovers OK. By the time I left she was waking up and the wound looked fine, so she should be all right, I think, but there's always the chance that the pin will back out or there'll be some other complication.

Monday 17 March

6.30 p.m. We had a superb weekend. We had nothing planned but then Greg, who's a friend from college, rang up and invited us down to Cornwall where he's working. Greg's into surfing as well and we went out on Saturday to a beach right down by Land's End. The surf wasn't fantastic but the water was so clean and clear it was amazing. In North Devon you can rarely see more that six inches into the murky sea, but there you could see the bottom as if it was only a few inches deep. It reminded me of surfing over coral reefs in Bali, where you can see the razor-sharp reef through the waves and it looks as though there's no water between you and it. The quality of the waves was nothing like Bali, but it was fun to be out there with only Greg and me in the line-up.

Emma walked the dogs along the beach while Greg and I surfed, and even got Pan to swim a bit. Badger is still too nervous to go in more than ankle-deep water.

Greg showed us the practice where he's working. It looks a bit like my place in that it's a converted house set in quite large grounds, and the inside is relatively old fashioned. The practice is mainly large animal, which is what Greg always used to like doing, but he was saying that he's getting more and more interested in small-animal work and wants to try to expand and improve that side of the practice. Apparently the standard of small-animal work is pretty low because the partners have always devoted most of their time and energy to large-animal work and haven't really kept the small-animal side up to date.

I told him about how it seemed to compare to Bideford. Although on the surface things seem similar in that the practices both used to be mainly large animal and are run by older vets, Witten Lodge has a more modern approach to small-animal work. I think that's due to Ian and Keith, who make quite an effort to keep up to date with modern techniques and developments. It's really Ian, although the older of the two, who tends to be the most interested in keeping the small-animal side of the practice up to date.

When I arrived at Witten Lodge, Ian was very keen for me to introduce any new techniques or ideas that I had into the practice. I think a lot of the older-fashioned practices tend to get a bit stuck in their ways until new, younger vets get to partner status, when they have the authority to make changes. Ian is always very receptive to new ideas and I think he sees the relationship between partner and new assistant as one where knowledge and ideas can flow in both directions.

Greg said that he's finding improving the standard of small-animal practice a challenge, but a bit frustrating as well, due to the attitude of his bosses, who seem to be fairly happy to let things plod along as they've always done. He's one of these people who gets really enthusiastic about an idea, so I can see him making some fairly big changes. I just hope he doesn't push himself too far and end up in a situation like I was last week with the leg pinning, or worse. Confidence is a great asset in vet work, but as I'm learning, overconfidence can be disastrous.

*

Something very strange happened on Sunday morning – we were all woken up by an earthquake! We had all had quite a lot to drink on Saturday night, so when the walls started to shake and everything was wobbling and creaking I thought for a second that it must be the mother of all hangovers kicking in, but as I woke up fully, I realized it must be an earthquake. It was all over in a few seconds and no damage was done, but it was a very strange experience. Until we saw confirmation on the news, we couldn't quite believe that it was actually an earthquake, but apparently it was, and it had its epicentre about fifty miles away, in the sea.

Today has been pretty routine. The cat that I pinned on Friday went home looking good, and Bonnie the bleeding bitch came in to have her stitches out. She was fine and Mrs Lawrence was relieved that it's all over; not, however, as relieved as I am!

Tuesday 18 March

Very dull day today. Morning surgery almost empty and only two people in afternoon surgery. There was only one farm call and Ian did that while I spayed two cats. While it was quiet I asked Ian about getting an X-ray developer and he said that he agreed and he'd talk to Keith and look into it.

I'm having the day off tomorrow to go on the nutrition course with Charles Moore, which should be quite interesting, and is better than another dull day of boosters and spays.

Wednesday 19 March

9.00 p.m. We got back about an hour ago after a good day out. The course was in Slimbridge Wildfowl Trust just north of Bristol. The place was amazing, there were thousands and thousands of water birds everywhere, with observatories to watch them from. None of the birds were captive, the Trust just provided lakes and nest areas for them and they returned year after year to what was water-bird heaven!

There were about a hundred people there, most of whom were farmers, although there were several vets as well. The talk was interesting and should be useful. They discussed the effect of feeding on fertility, a lot of which will be really relevant to most of our farmers, especially Charles, because he's having a problem with poor fertility in his newly calved cows.

On the way home in Charles's Land-Rover we ended up having a really long talk about vets and farmers and what's wrong with the way the system works at the moment. By the end of the journey we'd both come up with an idea about how to improve the service that farmers get from their vet, and the job satisfaction of the vet. What we decided was that the ideal situation would be if a group of farmers got together and employed their own vet, rather than going through an existing practice. The farmers would then get a dedicated vet and have no worries about vet's bills as they would all pay a lump sum each year to cover the vet's salary and expenses. The vet could then work entirely in the farmers' interests (or rather the farmers' animals' interests), as opposed to having to try and make money out of the farmers as one has to at the moment. I think this would be good for the vet as well, as you could really work with the farmers and improve the way their farms are run, without the ulterior motive of making money from it.

I suppose the only real problem would be that the vet would be on call all the time, and the farmers might abuse the system and continually call him out, if they didn't have to pay extra.

I shouldn't think that it'll happen, at least not for some time. I'm not even sure whether it'd be allowed by the Royal College. You never know, though, maybe in a couple of years I'll look into setting something up along these lines. I think

I need a little more experience before a group of farmers entrust their livelihoods to me completely!

Friday 21 March

I went over to Dulverton last night. Emma was on call, and she had to go out and see a cow at about 9 p.m. While she was out, the phone rang and, as I was there, I answered it rather than letting the answerphone get it. It was a woman who was really worried about her dog because it had been ill for some time and was now really bad. Apparently Emma had seen it that afternoon, but it was now worse and she wanted a visit as soon as possible. I said that Emma was out and that I'd get her to ring as soon as she got in. I didn't say I was a vet because I thought it would just complicate things.

Emma was gone for ages and I had no way of contacting her, so I was faced with a real dilemma when the lady rang back about twenty minutes later saying that the dog was worse and could someone come out quickly. I thought again about telling her I was a vet and going out to see her, but I thought I could get into so much trouble if something went wrong. If I'd gone out and the animal had died, I don't know what would have happened, because I didn't work there and knew nothing about the case. So I just said that Emma would come as soon as she could, and hoped she would get back soon.

She did get back about ten minutes later and went straight out to see the dog, but it died soon afterwards. Emma said she'd been treating it for a couple of weeks for a really nasty abscess and internal infection, and there was nothing that could have been done. I felt pretty bad that I'd not gone out, because even though Emma said nothing could be done, I still thought that maybe I should have at least tried, and that if someone had got there half an hour earlier, it may have been savable. I suppose that's just me being silly, really.

The more I think about it, the more I think I did the wrong thing. I swore an oath to look after animals, which I failed to keep. I shouldn't worry about the details of whether or not I might get sued or sacked, I should have had the welfare of the animal as my first priority. Next time, if there is one, I know what I should do.

It's a very difficult job at times. You have to make so many crucial decisions each day, and every now and then you're bound to get one wrong. So far in my career I've been lucky with my mistakes. Greg told me at the weekend that about one in seven vets get sued in their first year in practice, I just hope I'm not going to be one of them. He also said that 90 per cent of vets crash their practice car in their first year as well. I hope when my crash comes, if it does, that I get away with a minor bump into a lamp post rather than a head-on collision with a lorry or something. Maybe I should go out and drive very slowly into a wall so that will count as my crash and I won't have any more serious ones!

Saturday 22 March

11.30 a.m. Just finished morning surgery, which was OK. I saw leg-pinned cat, which is doing very well and starting to use the leg a little.

I was planning to go grassboarding this afternoon but I was messing around with it in the car park outside my house when it got out of control and hit next door but one's front porch. They weren't in, luckily, but it bent the axle so badly that it's completely unusable. I have a sneaking suspicion that Peter was right in the first place and rubber bushes would have been much better than a solid joint using springs. It's back to the drawing board!

Sunday 23 March

8.00 p.m. Dulverton Spent most of the weekend over at Emma's because she was on call. The lambing season is in full swing and she was really busy. I think she's enjoying a lot of the work but she said that she's getting pretty fed up with nasty lambings which the farmers have left too long and, as a result, the lambs are dead and often rotten. I get it o easy compared to her. This is roughly what she saw today:

> 7.45 a.m. lambing (two dead lambs)
> 9.00 a.m. visit to sick calves (diarrhoea, given fluids and antibiotics)
> 9.30 a.m. visit for lambing (one live lamb, one dead)
> 10.45 a.m. lambing (caesarean section, one live lamb, ewe fine)
> 1.00 p.m. vomiting dog (antibiotics, anti-inflammatory, anti-emetic)
> 3.00 p.m. lambing (two very dead and smelly lambs)
> 7.15 p.m. lambing (caesarean section, two live lambs, ewe fine)

She's just been called out to yet another lambing. I'd love to help, obviously, but I can't as I'm not employed by the practice, so I'll have to stay in and watch telly instead.

11.00 p.m. Serves me right! I was just getting into *Inspector Morse* when Emma rang and asked me to go out and help her. After the lambing, she'd had to go straight to a farm miles away across the moor to see some cows which had gorged themselves on straw. She'd decided that the worst of the cows needed an emergency operation to remove the food from its rumen as it had formed a serious impaction, and that it would be much easier with two vets. After what I'd done (or rather not done) last week with the sick dog, I didn't quibble about the ethics, and headed off to help.

It was absolutely freezing at the farm, with a Siberian

wind howling across the moor and into the barn where the cows were housed. Rain was splashing down through holes in the roof, making the whole experience extremely unpleasant. Emma said I was just soft because all my farms had nice weatherproof buildings and this was real, tough vetting!

She got on and opened up the stomach, with me assisting, and together we removed a massive pile of partly digested food. After a couple of hours bent over in the freezing conditions, we were both soaked and cold to the bone. It was worth it, though, because the op went well and should save the cow. The others weren't as badly affected and should cope without surgery.

Although we were both tired and cold, we felt a sense of real achievement – real 'fire-brigade' vet work. The satisfaction of saving an animal easily outweighed the discomforts and the missed *Inspector Morse*!

Monday 24 March

1.00 p.m. I completely forgot the BBC were coming this week, so it was a bit of a shock when I arrived at the practice to find Sarah and Emma, plus crew, waiting for me.

No exciting cases came in this morning so they just hung around and generally got in the way. The only cases they filmed were a mouse with a lump, which I put to sleep – so I shouldn't think they'll use it – and a cat with fleas, which is probably too boring. They didn't seem to mind too much, though, I suppose that's the way things like this go, you have to put up with lots of unproductive time to get the occasional exciting moment.

I've mended the grassboard so that it is usable again, so if there's nothing going on this afternoon, they are going to come and film me riding it, which should be amusing.

5.00 p.m. We took the grassboard out to a small hill nearby and they filmed me having a few runs. It was going fine and looking pretty good until I tried to turn a bit too sharply and fell over quite hard. I was OK, but the grassboard wasn't so lucky, the whole of one axle ripped off and continued down the slope on its own, with me sitting in a pile of thistles watching and being filmed. I felt quite embarrassed by the whole fiasco, I just hope that it doesn't make it to the final programme. My grassboarding empire could be finished before it's started!

Tuesday 25 March

Excellent day today. The BBC have got a really interesting story, and I got to do some good surgery.

It all started in morning surgery. I had just finished with a very sick hamster (finished in the final sense that it died while I was injecting it) when Sue ran in and said someone had just rushed in with a cat which had been attacked by a dog. I called the couple, Mr and Mrs Craner, through and they hurried in with their small ginger cat, Splodge.

''Ee's bin had be nex-door's terrier,' said Mr Craner in a gruff Bideford accent, which went with his gruff Bideford appearance. He had very short hair and a large scar running down one side of his face. Not a man I would want to pick a fight with, I thought as I lifted up the cat.

Just as I was starting to examine the cat, Sarah came in and asked if they could film the case. The Craners seemed not to mind, so the crew piled into the consulting room and started filming.

'Right, he's broken his jaw,' I said after a couple of minutes. 'See here where these two bits are moving, and here as well.' Splodge had in fact broken his lower jaw in two places, at the front in the mid-line, and right at the back on the left-hand side. 'He's also got some wounds on his chest, and I can hear air under the skin, which could be from his chest, but hopefully is just from these puncture wounds,' I added as I turned him over. 'What we'll do is have him in, take some X-rays to see exactly what he's done to his jaw, and check that his lungs and chest are OK. Assuming that his injuries are limited to what we can see now, we'll have to operate to wire his jaw back together.'

I was trying to maintain a cool professional exterior and not give away the fact that I was really excited by the prospect of fixing the jaw. I just hoped the X-rays showed no more injuries and the jaw fractures would be reasonably easy to mend.

The X-rays did show that, apart from the jaw, Splodge appeared to have been very lucky. The jaw, however, was more seriously damaged than I'd first thought. It was broken in two places as I'd suspected, but the second fracture was right at the back of the jaw, and would be quite a challenge to fix.

Not wanting to repeat the mistake of plunging in without assistance, like I had done with the leg pinning, I found Ian and asked for his advice.

'Yes, that's a tricky one,' he said, looking at the X-rays, 'the mid-line fracture should respond to wiring back together, but the other one is more of a problem.'

We consulted a surgery textbook and assessed the options. I was all for trying a technique shown in the book where you create a 'bumper bar external fixator', which consists of a curved bar positioned about one centimetre away from the jaw, with five or six pins locating the jaw fragments in place. Ian suggested a more cautious approach.

'No, no, that's asking for trouble. It's always better to rely on the animal's natural healing powers rather than barging in and making a mess of the situation. The best thing to do in this case is going to be to drill a hole in each fragment and join them with a loop of wire.'

In the end we did as he had suggested, working together. I was a little annoyed when he scrubbed up to help, because I'd wanted to do the op on my own, especially with the cameras there, but, as it turned out, he let me do most of it and just advised and helped where necessary.

The op took the best part of an hour, mainly because I'd never attempted anything like it before. It was a very strange experience using a normal Black and Decker drill (in a sterile drape) to drill into living bone. Once I'd got over the initial feeling of nervousness, I found it was really just the same as normal DIY. I think all the drilling I've done in making the grassboard has stood me in good stead! The end result was pretty good: the jaw was stable and as Splodge is such a young cat, it should heal well.

I was glad of Ian's help. If he'd not been there, I would have plunged in on my own and probably tried something far too complex and difficult, which could have ended in disaster. One of my failings is my overenthusiasm. In cases like this I'm always too keen to try new and exciting surgery without giving the consequences enough thought.

I had one bad experience soon after I qualified, when I tried a very tricky op on a cat. I made a real mess of it and left the cat much worse off than before I started. In the end it had to be put to sleep, although I think that would have happened regardless of what I'd done. It was another of those cases where, even though I made a real mess of it, the owners were lovely and thought I'd done the best I could. I felt like saying, 'Sue me! I've just made a massive mess of operating on your cat and I deserve to be punished, not thanked.'

The first year in practice seems to be a minefield of potential disasters, and so far I've trodden on quite a few mines but fortunately none have gone off. Some of my friends from college haven't been so lucky; at least two have been threatened with legal action already. One was because he operated on a very ill rabbit and saved its life but had not got specific permission from the owners to do the operation. It had got to the stage where he couldn't reach the owners to get their permission, but if he didn't operate immediately the rabbit was going to die. He decided to go ahead and the rabbit survived, but the owners were angry and threatened him with legal action for not consulting them before the op.

It does amaze me what some people will try and sue vets for. I'm sure that if the vet had not operated, the owners would have tried to sue him for negligence or something – there are just some clients who will try and blame someone for everything that happens and want to sue for any perceived wrongdoing or mistake.

Thursday 27 March

1.00 p.m. The BBC have just left, thank God. It's been good having them around and they got some good stories, but it gets a bit much after a while. They keep getting me to repeat things over and over; I feel like an actor more than a vet at the moment.

Splodge is looking OK. He's not really eaten anything yet, but he's pretty bright and alert so he should start eating soon. I hope we don't need to put a feeding tube down, because he really needs to start using the jaw to make it heal properly.

Yesterday the BBC filmed the Craners at home, and the offending dog next door. The next-door neighbours have offered to pay the bill, which is pretty good of them, considering the cat was in their garden and it wasn't a case of their dog escaping and attacking the cat.

Friday 28 March

Splodge is improving by the day. Last night he ate a small amount of liquidized food, and today he's eaten a big meal of soft cat food. His jaw is moving freely and there's no sign of any instability or discomfort, so he should be fine. I just hope he's learnt that Rex next door is not a dog to be messed with.

The next-door neighbour came in and paid the whole bill today, which came to just over £200. I think it was pretty reasonable considering it took two vets about an hour to do, plus the nurse, the drugs and the X-rays. People complain about vets' charges but if you compare them to something like garage bills or private medical bills, they're not too bad. I had to get some work done on my car when I was a student and for just having a few new parts, a couple of hours' labour and an MOT, it cost nearly £300, so I don't feel too bad about what we charge. Most people don't think about the potential costs of vet's bills when they get a pet, so it comes as a nasty shock if their animal has a serious problem. Pet insurance is the way forward I think, it's cheap and allows the owner to have their animal treated in the best way possible, and the vet to do his best without having to worry about how much it'll cost the owner.

Saturday 29 March

8.45 a.m. Oh no! The start of a whole weekend on call, and I'm due for a busy one by rights.

Pan has chewed one of the legs of the kitchen table overnight, the mutt. I've protected it from further gnawing by putting an empty plastic milk bottle round it. When I leave I'm going to have to run away to Brazil or somewhere to escape the wrath of Ian and Keith when they see the state of the practice house.

9.00 p.m. Busy, busy, busy! I've been on three calls since morning surgery, including one calving (fairly straight-forward) and one calf with a broken leg.

It was nice to get a relatively easy calving done, after what happened last time. This was in a nice warm, clean calving box full of fresh straw. The farmer brought me a big bucket of steaming hot water, and I even got soap and a towel and, to cap it all, a mug of coffee afterwards! It was a bit of a contrast to the battle in the trenches which was the calving where Ian had to come and help me a few weeks ago.

The calf with a broken leg was out at Ford's farm on the Torrington road. The farm has got a massive long drive, where I usually turf the dogs out to run alongside the car. They love chasing the car and can keep up when I'm doing nearly thirty miles an hour. As well as being a big dairy farm, the Fords also rear pheasants for the local shoot, and there are usually quite a few wandering around along the driveway. Until now I'd always managed to avoid them, but when I drove up to the farm today, disaster struck. As I was looking round to see where the dogs were, I heard a thud and felt a bump. I stopped the car and leapt out to see the very still form of a dead pheasant lying in the middle of the drive. I feel bad about what I did next, because I really should have picked the bird up, taken it back to the farm and admitted to Mr Ford what I'd done, but instead I hid the body in bushes and drove guiltily and cautiously on to the farm.

I'm not the greatest liar in the world at the best of times, so I found it very hard not to admit to my crime as I was talking to Mr Ford about the calf I was examining.

The calf had a broken back leg, just above the hock, so I decided it would probably heal reasonably well in a cast. I fetched some casting material from the car and applied a fibreglass cast around the leg. These modern materials are so much better than plaster of Paris. They're much lighter and stronger and easier to use as well.

We started chatting about a problem that he was having with infectious diarrhoea in calves reared in one of his sheds. Apparently lots of his calves were getting really bad diarrhoea after being moved to this one shed.

'What was in the shed before the calves?' I asked, and then immediately wished I hadn't.

'Oh, just them pheasants you passed on the way up 'ere,' he replied. 'We rear 'em in 'ere for the first couple of months before they're big enough to be let out. They're a great lot this year, very good birds, worth a bob or two as well.'

Oh no, I thought, not only have I mown down one of his prize birds and not admitted to it, but it looks like they might be involved in this calf problem. There's going to be a lot of pheasant talk, and I'm bound to let my terrible secret out. He'll probably demand compensation, report me to the Royal College, and tell Ian that he'll never have me back on the farm.

I managed to survive taking some samples and discussing the calf scour problem without giving anything away, but I was very relieved to drive off once we'd finished. I drove very carefully, with the dogs in the car, and managed to make it to the main road with no more kills on my conscience.

I just hope he doesn't do a head count (or beak count) this evening, or go rummaging in the bushes.

Monday 31 March

Played squash with Keith again last night and lost again. He might be twenty years my senior and a little overweight, but squash is one of those annoying games where skill matters more than youth. I might have to take up golf to see if I can beat him at that, although thinking about it, I'd rather lose at every sport in the world than take up golf.

Where I walk the dogs, on Northam Burrows, there's a golf course, and the golfers really make me laugh. They walk around in their diamond-pattern jumpers and check trousers, and spend three hours alternately digging holes in the ground with their clubs and fishing balls out of ditches. How much fun can that be?

Pan and Badger love golf balls, so quite often I'll be wandering along and turn round to see each dog chewing away on a golf ball. In the distance there'll be a group of irate golfers bashing their way through the brambles trying to find the missing balls, which by then are rapidly becoming unrecognizable dog chews.

Keith plays quite a lot of golf, and tends to spend many afternoons down on the course while I'm working. I suppose it's his right as he's the boss, but it doesn't exactly endear me to golfers in general.

Local people are allowed to keep animals on the Northam Burrows, so there's quite a few sheep wandering around. They tend to be pretty badly looked after because the grazing is free, so people think they can just buy a few animals, let them loose on the common ground, and they'll take care of themselves. When they do have problems, the owners either don't notice, or can't afford veterinary treatment, so the animals don't get seen to. The only time we see them is usually when someone walking on the Northam Burrows spots an injured or ill animal and rings us up. By the time we get there it's often gone, so it gets pretty frustrating.

I'm sure a few sheep are killed each year by stray golf balls as well, another reason to ban the barbaric sport!

April

Tuesday 1 April

1.00 p.m. Had to go out to the Fords' this morning and re-cast the calf's leg because it had somehow broken the cast. I put on a double thickness layer this time, so hopefully it won't break again.

We haven't had the results from the calves yet so I managed to avoid the subject of pheasants. When I drove up I was dreading Mr Ford meeting me with a grim face and a dead pheasant, but luckily he was still ignorant of my crime and was all smiles and jokes. How long can I keep up this charade?

10.00 p.m. Just finished speaking to Mum on the phone. She's suggested that me and Em go out in a couple of weeks. A week in the south of France sounds very appealing, but I'm not sure if Emma will be able to get the time off as her practice is so busy with lambing at the moment.

I haven't been out to see my mum since last summer so I should go fairly soon. While I was at university I managed to spend a couple of weeks a year with her, but since I've been working it's been a bit harder to find the time. I really missed not having her around when she first moved while I was in the first year at Bristol, but I suppose I've kind of got used to it now. It definitely has its good points, though, because she lives in a lovely little village about twenty miles from the Med, surrounded by vineyards with the Pyrenees in the background.

10.15 p.m. Just rang Em and she's going to ask if she can get the time off in a week or two. I really hope she can come because she's only met my mum once, and that was just briefly at graduation.

Wednesday 2 April

I had to visit Mrs Black over the road today. It's something that I've been trying to avoid for ages, because the nurses say she can be a little difficult at times, but there was no getting out of it today. Ian and Keith were both out and she asked for me specifically, even though she's never met me before. Sue told me that she latches on to a particular vet and won't see anyone else until she decides that one of the other vets is better for some reason.

She's got a massive Great Dane called Elly, which lives on its own sofa and very rarely moves. It's on regular monthly injections of steroids for its hips. At least I think it's for its hips, everyone just keeps on with the treatment, but I'm not entirely sure who diagnosed the problem or exactly what the problem is. It's one of those cases where it's better to carry on as before rather than upset things. I don't think that she has much of a life, cooped up inside all day, but she is about ten and that's pretty ancient for a Great Dane.

I turned up at about 12.30 after putting it off all morning, and the door was answered by Mrs Black. I think she's widowed because, apart from Elly and a couple of goats in the garden, she lives with her mother. She showed me through into the room where Elly was lying on a very worn and grimy sofa. The dog took very little notice as I injected the steroid into the muscle of her hind leg. I gave her a quick check over, but apart from being a little overweight and obviously arthritic in her back end, she seemed to be in reasonable health. That was more than could be said for Mrs Black, who was hobbling around with a stick.

'Rheumatism,' she explained. 'My hands are the worst, especially in the winter.'

'You could do with one of these injections,' I replied, joking.

'I have them, down at the hospital, when it gets really bad. I try to have as little as possible, because they're not good for you in the long term, are they? I know we've had Elly on them for years now but you should have seen her before – she could hardly walk poor thing. She's not done too bad either, ten's a pretty good age for a Dane, isn't it?'

I agreed. Most really big dog breeds tend to have pretty short life expectancies, sometimes as low as five or six years in some breeds, such as St Bernards. I think it's because they tend to be prone to lots of nasty problems, especially heart disease. If everyone just had nice mongrels (like Pan and Badger, who are dubious mixes of collie, pointer and a few unidentifiable other breeds) the canine world would be a much better place, if you ask me.

It was strange to see an owner suffering from exactly the same problem as her pet. I suppose at least she could really appreciate what pain the dog was in, and that's probably why she's kept having the steroid injections done. She knows that they work for her.

After I left I thought that although the nurses said that she could be a little difficult at times, she is actually quite a nice lady. The way she lives, in a messy, dirty old house, with the dog on the only comfy looking bit of furniture, is a little odd, but my only judgement should be on the health of her animals, not on anything else really.

I spoke to Ian about her when he got back and he seemed to have a bit of a soft spot for her, although he did say that he didn't really enjoy going into the house much. He said that she'd lived there for years and years and the house had gradually gone down hill ever since her husband died about five years ago.

Thursday 3 April

1.00 p.m. Had quite a busy morning doing farm work this morning. Ian is away in Austria visiting his in-laws. His second wife is an Austrian princess, so all the farmers keep telling me, but I'm not really sure if I believe them. Anyway, royalty or not, he's away until next week so I ended up doing all the visits (as Keith was busy with paperwork), which were:

Charles Moore (well run, efficient dairy farm) – 7
   scans, 4 fertility checks, 1 ill cow
Brown (another good dairy farm) – 1 wash out
   (very smelly), 3 fertility checks
Lake (smaller dairy farm, friendly farmer) – 12
   scans, 2 fertility checks, 1 casualty slaughter
   certificate
Bellew (very nice farmer, old-fashioned little farm)
   – coughing calves, 1 lame cow
Morris (first visit, small, grotty farm) – calving
   (easy)

8.30 p.m. Emma's over and she has said that she's managed to wangle a week off from the end of next week so we're going to go and spend a week at my mum's. I can't wait. It'll be so nice to get away from wet, grey and cold Devon for a while.

8.50 a.m. Just rang Mum, who's delighted that we're coming. She also said there might be a bit of vet work to do in the village because there's an old man with some cats, and one of them is in a terrible state. She said it needs its teeth looking at and the man is too old and poor to take it to the vet, so could we try and help when we come over? I said we'd have a look when we came, but there may be nothing we could do without taking it to the local vet.

Friday 4 April

We got the results from Ford's calves this morning, and it turns out that the pheasants are to blame. The calves are suffering from a rare strain of salmonella usually only found in game birds, and it looks very much as though they must have contracted it from the birds, which were in the shed before the calves.

I had to ring up Mr Ford to tell him, and I thought this would be as good a time as any to finally admit to my pheasant-murdering past. I was hoping that, as the birds were to blame for the problems with his calves, he wouldn't be too upset to find out that he was one bird worse off thanks to his trusted veterinary surgeon.

'Hello, Mr Ford? We've got the results from those calves of yours which were scouring,' I said.

'Oh, yes,' he replied. 'What's the problem then?'

'Salmonella from the pheasants. They've got a very unusual strain only found in game birds, normally, so it must have come from the birds. It should respond to antibiotics, but you'll have to make sure you don't spread it to the other calves. It would also be a good idea to keep the birds in a separate shed next year as well, if you can.'

While he replied that finding a different shed could be a problem, and that they might have to think about building a new one because they needed more space anyway, I plucked up the courage to tell him about my little accident. Finally, he finished rambling on about the new shed so I seized the opportunity and got it over with.

'I've got a bit of an admission to make,' I said. 'Last week when I was coming up the drive, I, er, accidently, er, hit one of your pheasants and, er, killed it. Look, I'm really sorry, I should have told you sooner, I'll pay for—'

'Oh, that's OK. Don't worry about it,' he interrupted. 'We've reared over a thousand this year and we always lose at least a hundred before the shoots start so don't worry about the odd one. They're a real menace on the driveway, aren't they? I think I've got at least three or four with the tractor.'

I was so relieved. I've been worrying about this all week, thinking I must tell him, and that he'd probably get really angry. I didn't realize quite how many birds they rear, I thought they might have had fifty or sixty at most, not over a thousand. I suppose it's no comfort to the one I hit, but one killed out of a thousand isn't quite as drastic as one in fifty.

I was going to be off all this weekend, but I've swapped with Keith so that I can have next weekend free and we can leave next Friday to go to France. That means I'm on tonight and all weekend, which is a bit of a pain, but it'll be worth it when I'm lounging around on the sun-soaked terrace sipping wine in a week's time.

Sunday 6 April

11.30 a.m. Just got back from walking Pan into Westward Ho! to get a paper and the ingredients for a fry-up. I'm not usually a fried food fan, but Sunday morning is a different matter – you can't beat egg, beans, sausage and bacon washed down with a gallon of tea at lunchtime on a Sunday.

11.45 a.m. Damn! This always happens, just putting the finishing touches to a fantastic-looking fry-up and the phone rings. It was Tony Fulford, who has got a sick cow, so at least it's not a 'drop everything and rush out' call and I can eat my food before I have to go.

11.49 a.m. Now feel very full and wish I hadn't eaten that extra sausage. Pan watched me eat the whole lot with a sorrowful expression as if to say, 'Pity poor Pan, for he is hungry.' He didn't get anything except one baked bean, which fell on to the floor.

12.55 p.m. Strange case that one. It's one of Tony's prize Jerseys, which calved about a month ago and has been off her food and ill for the last week or so. She looked very thin and in poor condition, but that can be quite normal in these heavy-milking dairy cows soon after calving. They can't eat enough to provide all the energy for producing the milk, so they have to use their body reserves to make up the difference. There, that nutrition course last month was worthwhile after all!

This cow was more than just in poor condition though. She was grunting in pain and had an elevated temperature. I couldn't find any obvious specific problem so I treated her with a painkiller and some antibiotics, and told Tony I would come back tomorrow to see how she's getting on.

I have a feeling she's got a fairly major internal problem of some form, so her outlook isn't fantastic. You never know, though, it may respond to the injections I gave her.

3.07 p.m. Got to go and see an old dog, possibly to put it to sleep.

4.00 p.m. What an emotional visit that was! It was an old man who lives down by the river in Bideford, and I've just had to put his beloved German shepherd to sleep. The owner was pretty distraught and wasn't making a lot of sense, so one of his neighbours was there to help him. In the end it was the neighbour who had to make the decision and sign the consent form, because the owner was too upset and confused. The dog was in quite a state and it was the best thing to do, but it really hit the old man badly. I suppose when you've had a pet for over ten years it must be like losing a member of the family when they finally go.

The actual putting to sleep went fine, which is always a relief, especially when the owners are so upset. The last thing you want in a situation like that is for it to take a long time and distress the animal.

9.17 p.m. Lambing!

9.55 p.m. Another of Mr Ashford's prize Suffolks with a fairly straightforward problem. He really reminds me of Richard Briers from *The Good Life*. Maybe it is him, and he's come down to Devon under an assumed name to escape from the media. I won't break his cover for him, but I might ask him discreetly about Felicity Kendal.

Monday 7 April

Went to see Tony Fulford's cow again this morning. It was no better really, and Tony was getting quite anxious to find out exactly what's going on. He's a fairly nice farmer, but he can be a bit awkward at times. His stockman is a really good bloke called Chutney and he seems to do most of the day-to-day running of the place and keeps it in good shape despite, rather than because of, Tony's input. I'm not really sure why Chutney is called Chutney, I've asked him but he keeps evading the question.

Chutney told me a few weeks ago that Tony is only really into farming as a sideline and that he made his money in business. As a result the farm doesn't actually make much money because he tends to spend all the income on new machinery and buildings. At the moment they're in the middle of having a massive new cowshed built, which is going to be amazing when it's finished. It will have top of the range cow cubicles, automatic muck scrapers, and is costing over £100,000, so Chutney says. I suppose it will be good for the animals, but I can't help feeling that the money could be better spent in other ways, such as improving their cattle-handling facilities.

Anyway, I'm pretty confused by this cow. She's obviously still in pain, but I can't see any reason why. She hasn't got mastitis, metritis or traumatic reticuloperitonitis. Her temperature is normal now, and she isn't lame. I took a blood sample to see if that shows up any abnormalities, but I'm not holding out any great hopes for a clear-cut answer from tests.

I don't want to fail with this one because I get the impression that Tony hasn't got total confidence in me and would prefer to have Ian or Keith out. I want to prove to him that I can treat and cure this problem, and then he may have more faith in me in the future. Unfortunately, this is bound to be one of those problems which are impossible to get to the bottom of, and it would be no different no matter who saw it. However, Tony would be much more likely to accept an admission of defeat from Ian or Keith with a feeling of confidence that all that could have been done had been done, than from the recently qualified young vet.

Tuesday 8 April

11.00 a.m. At last I've found something definite wrong with the mysterious Jersey cow. It's got a displaced fourth stomach. I had checked for this when I'd seen the cow before but was never convinced that it was the problem. Today, however, I heard a classic 'ping' under the stethoscope in a place which could only be the abomasum in the wrong place. I'm still not convinced that this is the main or sole problem because it shouldn't really cause this much pain, but I'm going to operate this afternoon to move the stomach back to its correct place and see if it does the trick. I just hope it does, because Tony is getting more and more worried and I can see he really wants to ask for one of the other vets. I probably should ask Ian or Keith to come and have a look, but I feel that if I'm right and I fix the problem, then I'll have not only saved the cow but won an important victory in the battle to impress Tony and bolstered my own self-confidence.

1.15 p.m. Well, everything went as planned. I took Taryn, one of the nurses, along to help and the operation seemed to go pretty much as planned. I'd never tried this operation on my own before so it was good to do it and for it to work, at least in the short term. Under local anaesthesia I made an incision on the right-hand side of the cow, where the stomach should normally lie. I then felt down under the large mass of the rumen and felt the inflated abomasum high up on the other side of the cow. Gently, so as not to damage the delicate tissue, I eased the stomach back under the rumen and let it float up into its correct position on the right-hand side. Then I stitched the stomach in place to prevent it moving back again, and closed up the incision. The whole operation took under an hour.

By the time I left, the cow was definitely brighter, but I still have a sneaking suspicion that the displaced stomach was secondary to some other more serious internal disorder.

I suppose I had no choice really, unless we decided to shoot the cow the stomach had to be operated on regardless of whatever else is going on inside.

Wednesday 9 April

I had to go over and see Mrs Black again today. It wasn't to see Elly, she's doing fine apparently, it was to see one of her pet goats, which is also lame. I think arthritis must be infectious in that household, because not only have the owner and the dog got bad joints but now it would seem that Muddy the goat is also suffering from the same ailment. The two goats, Muddy and Lucy, live in the garden. They've got a small goat-house for the night, but otherwise roam the small lawn freely. Muddy was obviously lame in one of her front legs when I approached, but despite this she was very difficult to catch and examine. Mrs Black tried her best but couldn't really help too much due to her own lameness, so I spent about ten minutes chasing the goat round the garden before eventually cornering her in the shrubbery and having a look at the leg. The problem was clear, her elbow was stiff and swollen, and she flinched as I flexed and extended it.

'It's either due to an injury, or it's infection in the joint, or it's just old age and wear and tear,' I said. 'Hopefully, it's due to a bang or something and a course of anti-inflammatories will clear it up, but if it's a chronic problem, she may need long-term treatment.'

I gave Mrs Black some sachets of an anti-inflammatory powder to give her, and injected Muddy with antibiotics in case there was any infection in the joint.

'I'll pop back in a few days and see how she's getting on,' I said as I left. I'm growing to almost enjoy visiting Mrs Black, even though it's a pretty grotty place. She's a genuine animal lover and looks after her pets probably better than she does herself, despite her disability. I just wish she'd get a cleaner in or something – the inside of the house is really grim. I suppose that cleanliness is not at the top of her priorities, and it would be a lot worse if she lived in a pristine, spotless house but didn't look after her animals.

Thursday 10 April

12.30 p.m. Saw the stomach cow out at Tony's today and she's not doing too badly. But she's still not eating very well and she's still grunting as if she's in pain, so something is still not right. Tony is concerned that I haven't solved the problem or, in fact, even found out exactly what the problem is, but he's happy with the op and how that's worked out, which is something.

I'll have to pass the case over to Ian now because we're off to France tomorrow. I just hope he agrees with what I've done, and when I get back she'll be OK and on the mend. If Ian immediately diagnoses something I've missed, Tony is going to be far from impressed with my performance. Vets generally have a code of practice where it is considered bad to disagree with another vet in front of a client. In some cases, though, there's no choice. If Ian finds an obvious problem he can't ignore it just to prevent me looking bad.

7.00 p.m. Mrs Johnson brought Jake into evening surgery for his annual booster. It was excellent to see him so bright and full of life. I had a good chat with Mrs Johnson, who said that he's been absolutely fine ever since the operation, but he hasn't learnt his lesson – they caught him trying to swallow an oven glove last week! I really hope he doesn't get anything else stuck, I don't think I could cope with the stress!

It was really nice to see an animal which wouldn't be here if it wasn't for our help (admittedly in Jake's case it was a bit of a close thing), and to think that being a vet really is important and worthwhile.

9.20 p.m. All packed and ready to go tomorrow. Pan knows something is up because his bed is all packed away to go to Emma's parents, who are looking after the dogs while we're away. He's sulking behind the sofa.

Friday 11 April

10.00 a.m. Dulverton Finally made it after getting on to the A39 and realizing I had forgotten to sort out Blackie. This is a cat which came with the house when I moved in. We don't get on at all well – I'm convinced that he is the devil in feline form because he is jet black and has the most evil stare I've ever seen in a cat. I'll be sitting on the sofa and I'll look round to find his unblinking yellow eyes fixed on me. I've tried to out-stare him but it's no good, I always have to look away first. I feed him when he's there but he wanders off for days at a time, he's probably out sacrificing small children or starting wars somewhere. Pan and Badger are scared of him as well, I think they can sense the evil spirit in him!

I asked the nice but slightly mad lady next door to feed him. She's the only neighbour with whom I'm still on good terms, and that's because she's very senile and deaf. The other neighbours have a list of grievances ranging from car parking offences to where and when I walk the dogs. I'm not sure if she really understood about Blackie, but I'm sure he'll survive on the blood of his sacrificial victims if she forgets to feed him!

April

2.30 p.m. Kent The dogs are very happy to be here. They've been to stay a few times and they love it. Penny, the family dog, is less keen on having them as visitors. She's a lovely old collie who's getting on for fourteen now, and she's pretty frail. Pan and Badger tried to boss her around when they first came here, but even though Penny is old and weak, she still put them in their place. Now they get on well together, and having them around seems to liven her up a bit. I think Emma, especially, finds it quite hard to see Penny getting old, because she was such an energetic, boisterous dog when she was younger and now she's very stiff and is going deaf and blind. It must be difficult to come home every few months and see her getting older and weaker each time. I suppose it'll happen to Pan and Badge eventually, but it's hard to imagine them as old and decrepit dogs, they're so full of life now. It only seems like yesterday we picked them out of the litter at the farm. I remember Pan so clearly – he was the big bossy kid of the class (he hasn't changed!) – whereas Badger was the shy tubby one hiding in the corner. I think we chose well, though, they're both excellent hounds.

I hope they behave themselves. Last time they stayed they chewed one of Emma's dad's gloves and dug a massive hole in the garden.

6.00 p.m. Gatwick In the bar waiting for the 8.05 to Toulouse. Emma's dad gave us a lift to the airport after an emotional farewell with Pan and Badger. I really miss them when we go away. I know they're just dogs but they've become so important to us it's hard to imagine life without their smelly licking faces following you around everywhere.

Midnight, Mum's house Here at last! Now to settle down for eight days of drinking too much wine, doing nothing and generally relaxing.

Sunday 20 April

7.00 p.m. Bideford What a fantastic week. We flew back yesterday and then stayed at Emma's parents' house last night. Pan and Badger were very happy to see us, and I think Emma's parents were pretty happy to see the back of Pan and Badger. They had completely destroyed the garden by digging two massive trenches at the top, and moving all the rocks and most of the plants from the rockery. They had also chewed the brand new coffee table and devoured a whole packet of hot cross buns which were on the work top in the kitchen. I think it may have to be kennels next time we go away.

We had a superb week in France, lots of wine and general lazing around. We didn't get away without some exercise, though, because Mum is a keen walker, and we got talked into one of her 'just a couple of miles round that hill' walks. This turned out to be a twelve-mile hike over a whole range of hills, climbing about a thousand feet in the process. It was worth the effort, though, because the scenery and the views were amazing. We found some wild mushrooms while on the walk, but we weren't sure which ones were safe to eat. On the way back towards the car, we came across a remote goat farm and Mum got chatting with the farmer, who told her which mushrooms we could eat and also suggested the best way to cook them. The goat farm was so different to anything in this country: the goats were roaming the hills searching the scrub and bushes for food, but came back to the farm twice a day to be milked. It's times like those that I really wish that my French was better. Mum speaks it fluently and I'm so envious of her. Every time I come here I go home with the resolution that I'm going to sit down and re-learn everything I was taught at school so that I could at least try to communicate. Emma and I love it over there, so it would be so much better if we could speak the language properly.

We've even thought about eventually moving to France one day.

The mushrooms were absolutely gorgeous when we ate them that evening, rounding off a really enjoyable and satisfying day. We felt we'd really earned our wine that evening – not that not earning it stopped us drinking it any other night!

I'm too tired to finish writing about everything we did, so I think I'll have a bath and carry on tomorrow. I wish I'd been bothered to keep up the diary while I was there, but I just felt like completely relaxing and not doing anything, so I failed to write a word.

I really, really wish that I didn't have to go to work tomorrow.

Monday 21 April

8.30 a.m. Oh, no! Work!

8.35 a.m. I wonder if Tony's cow is OK or not. I'd forgotten all about it until this morning, which is the sign of a good, relaxing holiday I suppose.

1.00 p.m. Busy morning back at work. Full morning surgery, which wasn't exactly what I needed to ease myself gently back into work mode, and then a couple of routine farm calls.

I asked Ian about Tony's cow and he said that it had been sent off to be slaughtered on Wednesday because it had really gone downhill. I was very disappointed. I'd thought that after I'd fixed the displaced stomach it would begin to improve. Ian also said he'd asked the slaughterman to have a look inside and see if there were any other things wrong which could have caused the problem, and he had found something else – there was a big abscess in the abdomen. It looked like it'd been caused by a penetrating object from the stomach, such as a nail or something, and that it had been brewing for some time.

This news made me feel a lot better because it meant that, although I'd missed something, it was something that would have been very hard to diagnose, and even if it had been diagnosed, treatment would have been near impossible. No wonder she was grunting in pain all the time and I couldn't find any specific cause.

I just hope Tony sees it that way. I think his only real justifiable criticism would be that I shouldn't have operated on the displaced stomach and that I should have sent her off for slaughter much earlier on. That's easy to see with hindsight, but at the time I didn't want to give up on the animal that easily. It's a bit like with small animals where you have to balance the chance of success against the cost to the owner.

However, I suppose you can say that a pet is a luxury item and you shouldn't own one unless you can afford to treat it properly if it gets ill, whereas a farmer makes his living from his animals and has to balance their welfare against his need to make them pay, to provide for him and his family.

8.35 p.m. Mum just rang to give me an update on the old man's cat. Apparently it's doing well now and the old man is really happy. This was the cat that she mentioned before we went over, with a very bad mouth. The man, who must be about seventy, lives in a tiny one up one down house round the corner from my mum in the village. He shares it with about three adult cats and a litter of kittens, who seem to use his bed as a nest. The house was in a real state: it stank, mainly of cats, and it really was like a nineteenth-century slum inside. The cats were all completely wild, especially the one that he said had the bad mouth. He told my mum it hadn't been eating properly for weeks and now it was pawing its mouth and racing around the house in pain, which are the typical symptoms of a nasty tooth problem.

Emma, Mum and I tried our best to corner the cat and catch it with a towel, but it was so wild and nasty that we had no chance. Emma got a nasty scratch on the hand before we had to admit defeat with the cat hissing at us from behind a dresser.

Back at Mum's house I decided our only hope of catching it would be to construct a device to snare it with, so we could then grab it and wrap it in a towel. From the store under the house I found a metal pole and some washing line and with these I managed to make a crude cat catcher, consisting of the pole with a loop of cord at one end which could be tightened. This is the basic design of the cat catchers we use at the practice to deal with particularly ferocious animals, so I knew it should work in theory without harming the cat unduly.

We all trooped back to the old man's house and had a second attempt. This time we were eventually successful, but not before the cat had knocked over most of the furniture in the room and scratched or bitten all of us. The final battle was fought out in a small space between the stairs and the dresser, with Emma distracting the cat using the pole and me looping the washing line around its neck. After a couple of attempts we finally caught it and managed to wrap it safely in a towel.

Once it was at least partially under control, we opened its mouth (using a spoon, which it almost bit through!) and briefly examined its teeth. They were in a terrible state, with several so rotten they were on the verge of falling out. The gums were badly inflamed and ulcerated, which was probably where most of the pain was coming from.

I told Mum, who relayed the information to the owner that the cat needed proper dental treatment under a general anaesthetic at the local vet. We'd brought some antibiotics with us, but without pulling the bad teeth out and cleaning the remaining ones, the tablets would have very little effect.

Mum rang the local vet and we booked an appointment

for the following day. We kept the cat in a basket overnight so as to avoid having to try and catch it again, and then dropped it off at the vet's the next morning, with a warning it might be a little troublesome. I was very glad it wasn't me that was going to give the anaesthetic!

When we picked it up later that day, to our amazement the vet not only still had all his fingers, but said it had behaved impeccably. Either he had some form of Gallic animal-charming skill, or he was lying to impress us! Either way he had pulled out the rotten fangs and cleaned up the rest. With the antibiotics, we felt that should be sufficient to completely sort out the problem. I suppose the only thing we didn't consider was quite how the old man was going to be able to give the cat the antibiotic tablets. We may have cured the cat but we also consigned the old man to a week of scratches and bites.

Mum did say he'd had a bit of trouble with the tablets initially, but since then he'd found that by wrapping them in a piece of goat's cheese, the cat came and ate them, no problem.

I hope it works out OK because he was landed with a bill for about £50 from the vet, which he really can't afford. I think Mum paid some of it and might end up paying the rest because he hasn't got a centime to his name.

Tuesday 22 April

Emma from the BBC rang last night and said that they want to come and film again next week. I almost enjoy having them come down now. The first couple of times was a bit unnerving and stressful, but now I feel pretty relaxed about being filmed, and they're such nice people that it's good fun most of the time.

They asked Ian to try and find some interesting characters or animals for them to film, so he's having a think about it. He did mention that there is a bloke in Westward Ho! with some parrots whose nails need trimming every now and then. He might give him a ring and see if we can go and do them.

Today has been quiet so I took the remains of the grassboard down to Peter and said he'd been right all along, and that rubber bushes were the way forward. I think the main reason it didn't work with springs was that it meant having a solid metal joint from the deck to the axles which would always be prone to breaking or bending. If we use rubber in between the board and the axle it will mean that there is a bit of give and flex in the joint so it shouldn't bend as easily. I described how I wanted it to work and said I would try and find some suitable rubber while he made the new axles.

I went back to the practice and had a look through the *Yellow Pages* for suppliers of rubber, and after a few embarrassing mistakes (there are a lot of different uses for rubber apparently!) I found a local supplier who could get me some suitable stuff.

I hope this idea works better than the last one. I'm sure the concept of a snowboard on grass will happen, it's just a matter of getting it right before someone else comes along and steals the idea. I'm going to look into getting a patent on the idea.

Wednesday 23 April

Had a dog in this morning that was castrated last week, while I was away, and now it's got a nasty hot swelling around the wound. I think it's probably just a bad tissue reaction to the surgery and the stitches, but it could be an infection, which may be serious. Its owners are a nice Scottish couple called Mr and Mrs McKenna, who are upset and worried by what's happened. I think I would be as well if Pan or Badger went in for a routine op and then a few days later ended up in real pain with a nasty complication.

It's a bit like the bitch spay nightmare I had the other

week, it's one of those things that can happen in any operation and it's usually just bad luck. In general we see very few post-operative complications, but with the number of operations we do each year, you're bound to get the occasional one with a problem like this. Saying that doesn't help the owners when it's their beloved animal with the nasty complication.

Although the McKennas were pretty upset, they were very understanding and didn't try to blame anyone. They were so worried by the dog, a little Cavalier King Charles spaniel called Toby, that they weren't concerned with why it had happened, they just wanted to get him well again. It shows that they are genuine people who really care about their dog. Some owners would have had their priorities the other way round, looking first to see who they could sue and blame and only then considering the animal and how best to resolve the problem.

Popped over to see Mrs Black this afternoon and she's very happy with how the goat is responding to the treatment. She was looking a bit more sprightly herself so I wonder if she's been trying the anti-inflammatory powder as well!

Thursday 24 April

8.15 a.m. I'm exhausted! I got called out at 10 p.m. last night to see a cat which was having kittens and it turned into a caesarean.

The owners of the cat run a small hotel up in Westward Ho! so when I arrived to examine the cat, I was surrounded by interested guests who wanted to see what was going on. After clearing the room of most of the unwanted onlookers (the owner's eight-year-old daughter steadfastly refused to go to bed as ordered by her parents and watched everything), I examined the cat, which had been straining without obvious effect for the last three or four hours. It was obvious that the kittens were alive and ready to be born as I could feel a tail wagging and a little foot moving with the tip of my finger, however the birth canal was too narrow to allow a natural delivery.

'We've got a couple of options,' I told Mrs Humphries, the worried-looking hotelier. 'We can either wait and see what happens or we can get on and do a caesarean on her. If we wait, there is a very slim possibility that she'll be able to kitten on her own or with a little help, but there is a more significant possibility that some of the kittens may die while we wait. If we get on with a caesar straight away we've got more chance of delivering all the kittens alive. If we wait and then have to do a caesar, she's going to be in a much worse state to take an anaesthetic, so the risk to her increases.'

Mr and Mrs Humphries exchanged glances and looked at their daughter.

'I think we'd better go for the operation,' Mrs Humphries said. Then added in a whisper so her daughter wouldn't hear, 'She wasn't supposed to get pregnant, so God knows what we're going to do with the kittens, we can't keep them here, but Sarah would be devastated if anything happened to Chloe.'

So, I took Chloe back to the surgery. The operation was the first caesarean I'd done on a cat but it was pretty straightforward and we delivered four live and healthy looking tabby kittens. There were no nurses around so I gave Chloe an injectable anaesthetic which I could reverse with a second injection once I'd finished. I also gave the kittens a tiny injection of the antidote to bring them around as the anaesthetic also affects them when they are in the womb.

Caesarean sections are quite straightforward operations really, much easier than a bitch spay for example. I think people have a misconception that routine neutering is easy 'do it with your hands behind your back' operating and that something more unusual like a caesar is much harder, and if something goes wrong it's more understandable.

By the time I'd finished it was after midnight. Chloe came round and immediately set to washing and cleaning the kittens. Mrs Humphries came down to the surgery and picked them all up.

'Four kittens!' she exclaimed in mock horror. 'What on earth are we going to do with them?'

I have my suspicions that if Sarah has anything to do with it they'll all stay at the hotel.

7.00 p.m. I saw Chloe and the kittens this afternoon and they are all doing fine. I asked Mrs Humphries what they were planning to do with them and she said they might keep at least one or two, and try and find homes for the others. I spot the devious influence of a young daughter at work! I bet by this time tomorrow she's convinced them that four kittens running around the hotel would actually be very good for business!

Friday 25 April

12.30 p.m. Mr McKenna came in this morning and I'm starting to get quite worried about Toby. The swelling has got worse and he's really in a lot of pain. There is also a rather nasty discharge oozing out from between the stitches, so I think it is more than just a tissue reaction and that there is some infection in there as well. I've put him on a really strong antibiotic and some painkillers which I hope will do the trick, because I don't quite know what we could do if they don't work. I suppose the only option is to open up the wound again and put in a surgical drain to help all the nasty infected material drain out. Whatever happens it must be horrible for Toby and is obviously distressing for the owners.

I've asked them to bring him back every day until we can get things under control.

6.00 p.m. Wonders will never cease. Keith finally got round to ordering the equipment for developing X-rays while I was away and it arrived this afternoon. We spent most of the afternoon after surgery had finished light-proofing the cellar so that we could use it as a dark room. Then we installed the safe red light and set up the tank into which we put developer, water and fixer in the three separate compartments. I was amazed how little there is to developing an X-ray, just two solutions with a water compartment to rinse the film in between the two, and that's it.

We took a test X-ray of a coat hanger and developed the very first Witten Lodge X-ray. It turned out surprisingly well, and took about ten minutes less time than it used to when you had to take it up to the hospital. It also means we will be able to X-ray emergency cases out of hours which could be life saving.

Saturday 26 April

9.15 a.m. Disaster! The developer tank is faulty and it leaked all over the floor during the night. The whole cellar is awash with highly toxic developing fluid. Keith is not happy: the tank alone apparently cost about £250 and it hasn't even lasted twenty-four hours.

10.30 a.m. Keith has managed to fix the leak with some industrial plastic cement so we are in business again. We refilled the tank and I'm just about to use it for the first time on a real diagnostic X-ray (lame dog).

10.45 a.m. Hooray! The film came out really well and showed, as suspected, that there is nothing seriously wrong with the dog's leg.

1.00 p.m. On call again thanks to my week off. I've just seen Mr McKenna and Toby. He's still bad, although he did eat this morning and he looks a little more cheerful. I think that's probably the effect of the painkillers rather than any great improvement in the actual problem. I've said I'll meet them at the surgery tomorrow morning for another check-up.

4.20 p.m. Milk fever at Philip Morris's farm. The cow responded well to the treatment and was up and walking around by the time I left. I got chatting to Philip about the BBC filming me and stuff, and it turns out that he's a bit of a TV man himself. Apparently he's been asked to feature in a documentary about Torrington and the Civil War because he's built a scale model of how the town used to look in the seventeenth century.

I really like Philip and his brother Steve over at Northdown farm. Steve is very different from Philip, he's very laid back about his farming and rarely calls the vet out, whereas Philip has regular visits and takes a much more serious approach.

I think the difference in their attitude proves to some degree the value of regular veterinary visits. In dairy farming the key to being profitable lies in minimizing the number of days each year that each cow is barren or not in calf. The number of 'barren days' is influenced by lots of factors, but the two most crucial are early and reliable pregnancy diagnosis and effective treatment of cows which aren't cycling properly. (It's always a disaster when your cows keep falling off their bicycles! Ha ha!)

This is where the vet comes in, and by having regular visits the farmer ensures that his cows are paying their way in the most productive manner. The vet can also ensure that the animals are being properly looked after and the farmer isn't sacrificing the welfare of his animals to increasing his profit margins.

Steve runs his farm well and the animals are generally well cared for, but his attitude of, 'Oh, she'll get in calf eventually,' or, 'She'll be right in a few days,' definitely leads to lower production and occasional cases where animals aren't treated as soon as they should be.

April

Sunday 27 April

8.00 p.m. Very quiet day so far. I went up to the surgery to see Toby McKenna and he's gradually improving. I suppose I should say 'the McKennas' dog, Toby', but I'm starting to get into the habit of giving long-standing animal cases their owner's surname. I think most vets end up referring to some of their clients like this, just for the sake of simplicity. It also helps to give the animal a bit more character. Rather than the animal being someone's property, like a car or something, it becomes an individual in its own right.

I also saw a sick cat (furballs) and a lame dog (thorn in pad), but apart from that it's not been too bad. I even managed to get a very quick surf in because Emma came over and she held the mobile phone while she walked the dogs on the headland. I tried out a little reef break off the headland called 'sewer pipe' by the locals, for obvious reasons. The break is directly out from the main sewage outfall from Westward Ho! and you have to time your surfing very carefully to avoid the times when they pump out the sewage, otherwise it gets pretty nasty! It's also a really shallow break over some sharp rocks, so if the tide is dropping it can get a bit dodgy, to say the least. Anyway, I survived both the threat of sewage and rocks and wasn't even called out, so it was quite a successful session really.

11.00 p.m. Still no more calls – I'm bound to get a 4 a.m. calving or something.

Blackie, the devil cat, has just dragged in a half-dead mouse, which I've confiscated and put out of its misery. Blackie gave me such a nasty death stare when I took his victim off him that I'm glad Emma's here tonight, I don't want to be alone with a disgruntled feline anti-Christ!

Monday 28 April

9.30 a.m. I was OK, no middle of the night call-outs, thankfully. I did have to go and see Mr McKenna at 8.00 this morning, though. Toby had had a really bad night and his swelling has got worse.

Mr McKenna looked tired and haggard when he opened the door.

'He's through here in the kitchen,' he said. 'Neither of us had a wink of sleep last night, he wouldn't settle and just kept moaning and whimpering. I almost called you out in the middle of the night, but I thought there wouldn't be much that you could do at four in the morning so I left it until now.'

I was very grateful for the consideration he'd shown, many an owner would have had no hesitation in ringing me up in the middle of the night, often for things much less important than this. In fact he was right, there would have been little else that could have been done if he had called me out, all I could have tried was a stronger painkiller, but I doubted whether it would have been very helpful. This was the kind of pain and discomfort which painkillers are worst at alleviating, the only way to stop it is to cure the problem.

Toby was pacing around the kitchen, obviously unwilling to lie on the swollen area underneath. When I lifted him up to look at the wound he yelped in pain and I could see the swelling was much worse and now looked very red and angry, with even more discharge from between the bulging sutures.

'I think we'll have to have him in and open the swelling up to try and get the infection to drain out. I don't think it's going to get better just on the antibiotics, and we can't leave him like this.'

'No, no we've got to do something,' agreed Mrs McKenna, who was on the verge of tears. 'He's in such a state, I just can't bear to see him like this any more.'

134

'I stayed up all night in the kitchen with him, and it was awful,' said her husband. 'I don't think I could go through another night like that.'

I really felt for them. Their trusting, faithful dog, who was really not much more than a puppy, was in such a bad state. To stay up all night, on the kitchen floor, really showed their dedication and love.

I don't think I've ever felt more determined to get a dog better.

Thankfully the BBC aren't coming until this afternoon, so I can get on with trying to get Toby better without having to worry about them. I don't suppose they'd want to film this case anyway, because they weren't in at the start of it.

11.45 a.m. Well, he survived the op, and I think what I've done should help his recovery. I re-opened the original wound and removed as much of the infected tissue as I could. Then I made the incision bigger and stitched in a piece of sterile rubber drain material to allow the infection to drain effectively. I closed most of the wound but left a hole at each end and sutured the drain in where it entered and exited. Hopefully, after a few days the swelling will be much smaller and, with the infection resolving, I can take the drain out and the wound will gradually heal up.

I've put him on the strongest antibiotic we've got. Now it's just a matter of wait and see how it goes, there's nothing else we can do if this doesn't do the trick.

7.15 p.m. The BBC turned up for afternoon surgery and filmed a couple of fairly dull cases. I wasn't on evening surgery so they couldn't film anything else. I felt as though they'd wasted their time a little. They were very lucky to be around when Splodge came in the other week so they can't grumble too much.

135

Tuesday 29 April

Ian has fixed up for us to go and visit Mr Jones and his Amazonian parrots this afternoon to clip their claws. It's mainly for the benefit of the BBC rather than any pressing need to do it. Ian said he usually goes and clips them every six months or so, and they'll really need doing in a couple of months' time, so it's not too much of a set up.

Apparently Mr Jones is a former high-society hairdresser, but moved down to Westward Ho! a few years ago to get away from the high-paced lifestyle of perms and tints, and now lives a quiet life in a bungalow near the sea. He sounds like an interesting character, and his parrots are supposed to be a little on the wild side – all the makings of a good BBC story!

4.00 p.m. Well, quite how I survived that experience without losing an eye or a finger I'm not sure. His bungalow is like a jungle, with parrots swooping at you from every angle. I had to keep ducking and dodging to avoid the flying hazards, and they weren't the only dangerous creatures in the house: he also has a couple of nasty little corgis, which kept nipping at my ankles.

Mr Jones is a nice enough person but a little strange. I suppose anyone who shares a house with four wild parrots and two man-eating corgis has to be a bit odd.

The actual clipping of the parrots' toenails was easy enough once we had caught them; it was the catching that was the problem. Ian and I spent about half an hour chasing the birds around the room, eventually cornering them one by one with a large towel. Once apprehended, one of us would try and hold the bird still through the towel, without losing a finger in the process, while the other clipped the claws.

The situation wasn't helped by Mr Jones' constant high-pitched cries of, 'Oh dear, do be careful, won't you?' and

'Oh, no, my poor little Topsy!' while we were grappling with his far from friendly birds.

The BBC were loving every moment, especially when Ian received a particularly nasty parrot bite on the finger, and when Mr Jones almost fainted from the stress of the whole situation.

I was worried that I would come across as being a bit incompetent, but I suppose that the series is there to document the realities of a first year in practice and the reality is that I've never tried to clip a parrot's claws before, so it's understandable that I would have a few problems. I think it'll probably just come across as quite funny rather than as bad practice or anything negative like that.

Wednesday 30 April

12.45 p.m. The McKennas brought Toby in this morning and I think he really has turned the corner. He was much brighter and more alert, and the wound is draining well from the tube I put in on Monday. Mrs McKenna said he ate most of his breakfast this morning, which is the first time in over a week that he's shown any real interest in his food. I told them we'd leave the drain in until Friday and then remove it, which we should be able to do in the consulting room without an anaesthetic, because it's only held in place by a couple of stitches.

They were both still looking tired, but were very relieved by what I told them; I really think he should pull through now. I was beginning to doubt whether he would a few days ago, but since we re-operated on him he's really started to improve dramatically.

Apart from that, the morning has been pretty quiet. The BBC crew came and filmed me trimming a couple of cows' feet at Brian Hill's farm. It was pretty unpleasant as usual, and in the end they didn't bother to film much.

7.20 p.m. Busy evening surgery. The BBC filmed an ill Labrador, an itchy cat and a Jack Russell with bad teeth. I don't think any of them will end up as suitable cases for the programme but at least they had something to film. Sarah, the director, said that just getting the one usable case, the parrots, was more than enough for three days' filming. Quite often they could film for three or four days and not get anything worth using, so they were happy with what they'd got this time round.

They're taking Emma and me out for another meal tonight to keep us enthusiastic about having them around. A free meal always does the trick for us – we'll do anything for a large steak and a couple of pints!

May

Thursday 1 May

Splodge, the cat with the jaw we wired back in March, came back in this morning. He's been having really bad breath for a week or so and now he's not really eating properly. My first concern was that the jaw hadn't set properly and was still unstable or infected, but when I opened his mouth I could see that although the jaw was solidly mended, one little fragment of bone was hanging loose. This little piece had trapped some food between it and the tooth, which was causing the smell, and where it was rubbing on the gum an ulcer had formed, which was responsible for the pain and lack of appetite.

In order to remove the bone fragment, I had to knock him out and cut one of the wires out which was holding it in place. I was a little worried that as I cut the wire the whole jaw would fall apart, but luckily only the loose piece came away and the rest of the jaw remained firmly fixed. As soon as the fragment was removed all the smelly food came away and it looked much more healthy. I was very relieved that our repair had worked and it wasn't a failure. It's quite common for metal implants such as wires to have to be removed after a while because of complications like this, so I still think I can consider the op to be a success.

Until he went off his food this week, he's been doing really well apparently and was pretty much back to his normal self. The only difference being that he's well and truly learnt his lesson about next door's dog and doesn't stray anyway near their garden anymore! Hopefully, this will be the last time we need to see him, the other wires which were put in can stay in place unless they cause problems later on. I don't think they will, because they're much more deeply embedded in the mouth and shouldn't interfere with his eating at all.

This case made me think about Emma, because she had an operation on her foot years and years ago, and had a metal screw put in. For ages it was fine, but over the last couple of years it has really started hurting. She's on a waiting list to have it removed, but it looks like it's going to be at least a year or more before she can have it done. I suggested that she should let me do it under a bit of local anaesthetic, I've got a screwdriver in my tool box somewhere. Surprisingly she didn't seem too keen on the idea and said she'd rather wait ten years than have me operate on her!

I can't see how operating on a human would be any harder than on an animal. If I can do complex internal soft-tissue surgery on a dog, such as a bitch spay, I should be able to do most basic human surgery. I think in emergency situations, vets are allowed to treat and even operate on humans, whereas doctors are not allowed to treat animals, even in emergencies. I'm not sure if that is true or just one of those long-lived myths that everyone passes on, like the fact that everyone seems to think that training as a vet takes seven years as opposed to five for a doctor (which it doesn't; it's the same – five years). That, and the old, 'Oh it must be so hard what with the animals not being able to tell you what's wrong,' are the two most common, and thus annoying, statements made by semi-interested relatives and people trying to make polite conversation.

I heard another dubious statistic the other day which is that of a poll of people asked the question, 'If you were climbing Everest and halfway up you developed a severe surgical problem which needed an emergency operation, who would you want to perform the operation, a GP or a vet?' The overwhelming majority opted for the vet. I suppose that's sensible because most vets have done a lot more operating that your average GP.

Maybe I should set up a little private surgical clinic in the practice at night when Ian and Keith aren't in, and do routine surgery at discount prices for people!

Friday 2 May

8.35 a.m. I must write this down. While I was lying in bed last night thinking about vets and operating on people and things, I had an excellent idea for a book. I've always wanted to write a book but never got around to it, but now I've thought of an idea I should have a go.

The basic plot is this: young, newly qualified vet fresh out of vet school arrives in remote country practice to start first job. However, at the practice, one of the vets is up to no good. He and his evil helpers are kidnapping innocent victims from the local town and taking them back to the surgery late at night where he anaesthetizes them and removes one of their kidneys. The kidneys are then sold to rich criminals who need transplants but can't find suitable donors, or can't wait for one. Our young hero discovers the fiendish plot and, in a final showdown in the operating theatre, defeats the evil vet. A bestseller waiting to be written I reckon!

1.20 p.m. Busy morning surgery followed by three routine farm visits.

1.25 p.m. Why would the practice employ the new vet if they were all in on the evil plot? Surely they wouldn't want to risk someone coming in and discovering what was going on? Perhaps . . . ah, yes! The old senior partner is unaware of the evil plotting of the younger partner and hires the new vet because he wants to think about retiring. The younger partner, or perhaps just an older assistant, is against the new vet coming, and does his best to get rid of him. He could sabotage his cases and make him look bad so the old vet will fire him. Of course, just before this happens our hero discovers what's going on and he reveals all to the old vet and all is saved.

4.00 p.m. The McKennas brought Toby in to have his drain removed this afternoon. He is looking excellent, the swelling is almost gone and he is so much brighter in himself. Even Mr McKenna looked as though he'd had a decent night's sleep. I asked him if he was still sleeping in the kitchen and he said that he had been but tonight he was going back to bed. Mrs McKenna looked pleased!

The drain came out, no problem, Toby hardly flinched. Now it's out, the holes should close over and everything should heal up fine. I am so glad he's OK. It's one thing to have an animal in pain and very ill after major surgery or a severe illness, but it's not what you expect after a routine operation like castration. It just shows that there are risks with all ops and you can never 100 per cent guarantee that things will turn out as they should.

8.00 p.m. Right! Pen, paper, no distractions, time to start the book!

8.35 p.m. I think Pan needs a walk. I'm doing pretty well, if a little slowly. I suppose one can't expect it to write itself. It's going to take a bit of effort.

> *The wind howled through the trees as Ben pulled up outside the imposing front door of the large Victorian house. Stepping out of the battered old Ford, he read the fading bronze plate to the right of the entrance, Harry Norton BVSc MRCVS Senior Partner.*

I've spent most of the last half an hour trying to think of the name for the evil assistant, so that I can add it to the fading bronze nameplate. The possibilities are:

Anthony Crabb
Damien Smith (too *Omen*esque)
Sylvester something
Keith (that has certainly got possibilities, although

I'm not sure Keith would be too impressed if I
named my villain after him)
Peter Crabb (for some reason I think Crabb is a
particularly evil surname)

9.10 p.m. Peter Crabb it is. Right, I'm going to sit down and
get a chapter or two done, it can't be that difficult.

Saturday 3 May

8.15 a.m. Just read what I wrote last night. I think it's going
reasonably well, although I only got as far as Ben (no
surname yet) reading the nameplate and being buffeted by
the storm. I'm not quite sure what he's going to do next, I
think I'll just let the plot flow and see what happens.

12.30 p.m. Very busy morning surgery again. It was particularly bad because it's a Bank Holiday weekend so everyone
wanted to get things out of the way before going off cara-
vaning or what ever they're doing.

I'm on call today and Sunday but Keith takes over on
Monday morning, thankfully.

Sunday 4 May

3.00 p.m. Just got back from taking Pan round the headland.
While we were walking back along the top of the cliffs he
ran up to a little collie. The owner asked if I could keep Pan
away because his dog was feeling a bit fragile.

'He's just fallen off the cliffs,' he said, pointing to the
drop a few feet away. 'He wasn't watching where he was
going and he just ran off the edge.'

'Bloody hell!' I exclaimed. 'That must be at least 150 feet
down to the beach.'

'Yes I know,' he replied. 'I thought he was a gonner, but
when I looked over the edge he was lying on the beach,
but he was moving. By the time I got down to him he was

walking about, and now he seems a bit dazed but otherwise he looks OK. I'm taking him up the vet to get him checked over just to make sure though.'

I explained that I was a vet and offered to have a look. As the owner had said, apart from being a little confused and disorientated, the dog was fine. No broken bones, no dislocations, nothing.

'That's amazing. To fall that far, bouncing down the cliffs, and not just be alive but to get away with no broken bones. It's incredible. Keep a close eye on him and bring him straight up to the surgery if he shows any signs of pain, or if the disorientation worsens, or if you're concerned at all.'

He said he'd bring him up if he was worried and thanked me for helping. As I watched him walk off, with the dog trotting along behind, I thought how amazingly lucky it had been to survive the fall. The cliffs are nearly vertical, and he'd landed on a hard shingle beach. I suppose he must have been unconscious so that all his muscles were relaxed, but even so it was a pretty amazing story. Perhaps I can incorporate it in the novel – Ben's loyal collie is lured off the cliffs by Peter because he's leading Ben to the place in the garden where the bodies of the victims who didn't survive the kidney-removal operation are buried!

Monday 5 May

8.45 a.m. Hooray! Phones transferred to Keith, back to bed!

10.15 a.m. Toby (friend, not the McKennas' dog!) has just rung up to say that he and Louise are coming over this afternoon to go surfing and go out this evening. The surf is looking pretty good, it's about three to four feet and fairly clean so we should have a good session. Emma's coming over in a minute so maybe I'll be able to get her to go in again. Although, knowing her, she'll go and sit in the pub all afternoon instead.

6.00 p.m. Excellent surf. Now off to the pub. I told them all about my book, but they weren't overly enthusiastic about the idea. I'll show them when I'm a rich, published author! That reminds me, I must go and see how Peter Bullock is getting on with the grassboard. He should have just about finished the new prototype by now. I picked up some rubber to make the bushes out of from the place I found in Barnstaple last week, so I may be up and riding again pretty soon. I told Toby about how it was coming on, and he seemed quite excited and keen to try it out, but he obviously still doesn't really believe it'll work.

12.30 a.m. Tuesday. Vewy good night, hic!

12.35 a.m. Oh no! Hic. Tobe's found whisky, I'm doomed!

1.45 a.m. Must go bed now. No more surf videos.

2.15 a.m. Bugger!

Tuesday 6 May

8.30 a.m. #&#@!!

9.00 p.m. Today not really worth writing about. This morning was spent in a hungover haze, and this afternoon was spent in a gloomy post-hangover-slightly-nauseous haze.

Wednesday 7 May

I had a sad case this morning. I had to go out to a house just outside Bideford and put a pet goat to sleep. I've never had to do this before, and it was strange to be treating a farm animal in the same way as a pet cat or dog.

The elderly couple who owned the goat kept her in a small shed at the top of their large, steep back garden. During the day she was allowed out to roam the garden, and was treated with more care and attention than a lot of small animals. As a result she had reached the ripe old age of fifteen, but over the last few months her back legs had developed severe arthritis and she was losing condition fast. She could no longer lie down comfortably or reach down to graze so, rather than prolong her obvious suffering, Mr and Mrs Humphries decided it would be kindest to have her put to sleep.

The injection worked very quickly and she died peacefully and without any fuss, which is always a relief. Mr Humphries had dug a grave all ready for her so I left the body with them. They were more upset over the loss of their goat than most people are when they lose a dog or a cat, but I suppose it's not really surprising because she'd been a loyal pet for so long and filled the same role as any other pet.

It's strange what animals people choose to keep as pets. Cats and dogs are well domesticated and make good pets most of the time, but animals like rabbits and pigs and birds are different. Rabbits can be quite good pets but I can't help feeling that in the wild they are naturally timid and shy and spend their lives trying to avoid predators, so it's a bit unfair to expect them to adapt to being a captive amusement for a loud child. They tend to suffer quite badly in terms of medical problems related to how they are kept, especially from bad teeth. This is mainly due to incorrect feeding and insufficient sunlight, and leads to horrible tooth abscesses, which can end up being fatal.

Pigs are also kept as pets sometimes, especially pot-bellied ones, and although they are probably much happier in captivity than some animals, they still tend to suffer from bad husbandry. People don't realize what they are taking on when they get a little piglet. A year later, when the cuddly little piglet has become a ten-stone, five-foot-long adult pig which is eating the flowerbeds and scaring off the neighbours, people start to have second thoughts.

Captive birds are one real dislike of mine. I can't stand seeing beautiful little birds cooped up in tiny cages with no room to fly, no other birds for company and nothing to do all day. I can't understand why people want to confine a creature to a little cage when it's designed to fly around the jungle. I feel really sorry for the birds, especially when they're brought in to the surgery because they've lost all their feathers. The owners are convinced that it's mites or something, but in 99 per cent of cases it's due to self-mutilation because they're bored.

Horses are similar. People lock them up in a stable all day, away from other horses, and then wonder why they develop strange behavioural problems like head weaving and repeated biting of the stable door. Horses are naturally herd animals and hate being kept on their own away from contact with other horses. The worst thing is that the owners of horses with these behavioural problems don't try to resolve the cause behind them (boredom, stress, anxiety, etc.), they just try to stop the horse's behaviour by putting bars across the stable door and things. This just makes the problem worse because the horse is then prevented from doing this stress-relieving action and then either does something new or bottles it all up inside and gets more stressed and unhappy.

It's the same as zoo animals. I remember Emma telling me that she was really upset when she went to a zoo as a child because she saw the polar bears, which were confined to a small, sterile enclosure, pacing repeatedly back and forth across the pen all day long. They had this stereotypic behaviour because they had nothing else to do and were so bored and unhappy they developed this strange repetitive action as a result.

I think zoos are getting better and are trying to give the animals more interesting enclosures which are more like their natural habitat, and this is helping to prevent the animals suffering, like the polar bears were. However, there are still millions of privately owned animals who suffer this kind of mental illness due to uncaring or just uneducated owners.

Thursday 8 May

2.00 p.m. Interesting, if somewhat gruesome, case this morning. I had to go and see a couple of calves out at Mr Hatherley's farm on the other side of Hartland, which he had described over the phone as having 'great big knackers on 'em'. I took this to mean that they needed castrating, but when I arrived and started to get my stuff out of the car he stopped me.

'No, I've already done 'em, but they've got summat there and ah don't know what it is like, come an' 'ave a look.'

He took me down to the calf-house and showed me the two calves. Both were about three months old and looked in pretty good health. However, when he caught hold of one and I looked underneath I could see there was something very wrong. Its scrotum was horribly distended to the size of a grapefruit and tapered in at the top to a very narrow neck where I could just make out the orange colour of a rubber ring. The other calf was in the same state.

'When did you castrate these calves, Mr Hatherley?' I asked.

'Oh, a month or so ago I suppose,' he replied. 'I know I shouldn't use the rings at that age but they always work well an' they're a damn sight cheaper than you lot.'

He'd tried to castrate the calves using rubber rings, which are placed around the neck of the scrotum to cut off the blood supply to the testicles. They should only be used in the first day or two of life because after that the testicles are too big, and the calf too aware of the pain. By using them a month after the calves were born, he'd caused them a great deal of pain and they'd ended up with what appeared to be large scrotal abscesses.

'I'll have to sedate them and try and sort out the mess,' I told him looking at the second calf, whose abscess was even larger than the first one.

In the end it took me over an hour to sort them out, and

cost the farmer about £150, roughly ten times the cost of castrating two calves. When I investigated, I found that what had happened was that he'd missed the testicles altogether and they were still there, above the rings. As a result, the scrotum had become necrotic and formed an abscess, which had slowly got bigger and bigger over the last month. I removed the infected tissue and castrated the calves, who were deeply sedated, having been given local anaesthesia. With a good course of antibiotics they should be OK, and it might teach Mr Hatherley a lesson in not cutting corners and treating his animals properly.

I always feel a bit self-conscious when I have to criticize or reprimand a farmer or small-animal client for doing something wrong. I think they're not going to take any notice of a young person like me, but they usually do. I suppose it's because I'm more used to being a student who nobody has any respect for! It is important to tell people if they are doing things wrong because in most cases of poor animal welfare, the cause is ignorance rather than anything more sinister.

Friday 9 May

I popped in to see Peter Bullock yesterday afternoon and he'd finished the axles for grassboard MkV or whatever I'm up to now. They're just what I had envisaged, and as soon as I assembled the board, complete with the rubber bushes, I knew that it was a vast improvement over the last effort. I tried it out on the park in Bideford today and it is fantastic, so much better than before. I think the next step is to use it as much as possible and see what it can do, and then try and get a video made so I can show it to potential investors.

As it was so quiet this afternoon, I went home for a while and tried to get on with the novel. I sat there for about an hour but in the end all I wrote was about half a page because I spent the rest of the time either re-writing what I'd done or sitting staring into space. I was quite pleased with what I did write, though. This follows on from what I wrote last week, where I'd got Ben into the lonely old practice looking for the senior partner.

> *The hallway stretched off into the gloom, illuminated only by one dim bare bulb near the front door. Ben cautiously moved down the hall until he stopped suddenly by a door marked Waiting Room. A man's voice was just audible from the back of the building.*
>
> *'Who the hell is that?' came the angry sounding enquiry. 'Don't you realize we close at six?'*
>
> *At that point the speaker strode into view, pulling off a pair of surgical gloves which, like the green surgical gown that covered most of his body, were stained with blood.*
>
> *He was a tall, gaunt man of about thirty years of age. His receding hairline was in contrast to a large bushy black beard.*
>
> *'Well?' he asked, obviously far from pleased to be interrupted. 'What's the problem?'*
>
> *'Er, well, er, I'm Ben, the new vet,' ventured Ben, rather unsure of whether it would be polite to proffer a hand or not.*

Obviously the evil assistant has been interrupted mid evil operation, but of course Ben will only realize the significance of what he's seen later on when he'll tell his new love (a vet nurse perhaps?).

> *'I was so stupid. It was him all along. I remember when I first arrived here, although it seems like a lifetime now, I was met by Peter, who was in the middle of an operation. I assumed that it was a dog or cat, but it must have been Davis or McDonald, or one of the others.'*

Then, with her help, he'll catch Peter red-handed and piece the whole plot together. I think it might end with old Mr Norton asking him to become a partner, and possibly marrying the beloved nurse (Elizabeth, Liz?).

Saturday 10 May

12.30 p.m. On this morning, but then off for the rest of the weekend. I went to see Mr Hatherley's calves after morning surgery and they're doing really well. I think he's been very lucky really. He promised that he's going to get us to castrate his calves in future, so it looks like he's learnt his lesson.

Toby's invited lots of people over to his house in Bridgwater tonight so Emma and I are going off there later on. It'll be good to see Tom and Pat and everyone else. It's been a bit of a change, leaving university and moving to a small country town where I don't know anyone. At university there were always lots of people around and we had a really good, busy social life, whereas now Emma and me tend to just see each other, and occasionally go and see friends like Toby and Tom. I suppose it makes you realize who your true friends really are, and who you spent time with just because you were all thrown together at college. Now we make the effort just to go and see people who we really want to see and, although our circle of friends is getting smaller, we've realized it's quality not quantity that counts.

Monday 12 May

Excellent weekend. We had a great time at Toby's on Saturday, and then on Sunday everyone came up here and we went surfing.

When we arrived, Toby had to pop into his practice to pick up something for his cat, so Emma and I went along to have a look, because he's always going on about how wonderful and modern the place is. I must admit that I was pretty impressed. It's a big, purpose-built surgery on an industrial estate, very different to Witten Lodge. Inside it's all very hygienic and sterile, with positive-pressure ventilation (so all the bugs get blown out of the building). There are two operating theatres, one for dirty operations like dentals, where sterility is not so essential, and one super sterile one for internal operations. They've got all sorts of fancy equipment such as endoscopes, blood machines, an ECG machine and an ultrasound machine, and everything is shiny and new.

It would be a great place to work from a professional point of view because you could really go to town on the cases and do everything properly without compromising too much. On the other hand, Toby has to work much harder than I do, and is rarely home before seven o'clock at night. He doesn't get the occasional two-hour lunch breaks and odd hour off in the afternoon that I get either. I'm happy enough where I'm working, and I'm not sure that I'd really want to work somewhere like that because it's all very high-powered and stressful compared to the relaxed pace of life in North Devon.

Tuesday 13 May

7.00 p.m. Off to Dulverton for the last pool match of the season. Pretty boring day today, lots of routine farm calls. Did see Mr and Mrs Gemmill when I was driving through Hartland so I stopped for a chat. They've just got a new dog, a ten-year-old terrier, from the animal rescue place over at Ilfracombe. They thought that a young dog might outlive them so they've taken on this lovely old dog. Apparently she was abandoned when her old owners went abroad. They had her with them, on a lead, so I had a quick check over and she looks fine. I hope she doesn't have any problems, because they went through enough heartache with Laddie.

Wednesday 14 May

7.45 a.m. Dulverton Oh, bad head! We were beaten at pool again last night, but it was good fun. Pan came very close to losing an eye from a stray dart as he was guarding the dart board, the silly mutt!

1.00 p.m. Calving at Philip Morris's this morning. It wasn't too hard but I managed to string out the visit so I made sure I didn't get back in time for morning surgery. I told Philip about the grassboard and he seemed really keen, so I asked him if I could try it out on one of his fields. He's got a beautiful sloping field across the road from the farm which looks ideal, and he said that it'd be fine for me to grassboard in it, and he also said that he might even be tempted to have a go himself.

I felt a bit hesitant about asking him to begin with because he's one of our clients and I should be acting in a professional and responsible manner, not asking if I can try out my new toy in his fields. In a way, although vets have to appear professional and serious, it's more acceptable to be a little eccentric and unprofessional occasionally than it would be in other jobs such as a bank manager or a doctor for example. People expect vets to be a little unconventional, it's all part of the mystique of our profession! Just look at some of the older country vets in their tweed jackets and classic cars – they're far from normal members of the community!

6.30 p.m. Just finished evening surgery and I'm on call. I can feel a busy evening coming on, because I've been much too lucky recently. The last couple of week nights I've been on I've not even had any calls, let alone visits to do, so I'm due a 3 a.m. calving or something.

7.40 p.m. I knew it. I was just settling down to carry on with the book (Ben has been shown to his flat above the practice by evil Peter, who has hurriedly finished off his dastardly operation out the back of the practice), when the phone rang. It's a possible put-to-sleep of an old dog.

Thursday 15 May

Last night was awful. The call-out I had turned out to be the worst, most stressful putting to sleep I've ever done.

I turned up at the practice and met the client, who was a middle-aged woman called Mrs Young, with her elderly Yorkshire terrier. I took her through into the consulting room and discussed the dog's various problems and looked him over. It was clear that she had come to the decision to have him put to sleep, and I agreed with her that it was the best thing to do. He was very old, incontinent, deaf and hadn't eaten properly for weeks.

Yorkshire terriers are not the easiest animals to find veins in at the best of times due to their size and the shape of their legs, and this one was even harder because of his age and weak circulation. Even so, the whole procedure would have been relatively quick and painless if it hadn't been for Mrs Young becoming more and more hysterical as I tried to find the vein. Each time the dog made a small yelp or wriggled she would cry out and accuse me of being unnecessarily cruel.

'Oh, stop, stop. You're hurting him! Oh, my poor little baby,' she wailed, moving the dog so that I missed the vein again.

After a couple of attempts she became more and more abusive, claiming that I was incompetent and probably only a trainee vet, and asking were there any senior vets around to take over because I was causing her little baby so much distress. I tried to explain calmly that if she would just let me get on with it without getting in the way it would all be over much more quickly. The main reason that the dog was getting upset was that she was so hysterical. If she would have just calmed down, or left the room, the whole thing would have been over in minutes, but she insisted on cradling

156

him in her arms and moving him away every time he flinched as the needle went in. Eventually after about ten minutes I decided the only option was to sedate him because by this stage he had become pretty distressed.

'I'm going to give him a little sedative to calm him down,' I told Mrs Young.

She agreed, but still persisted in questioning my ability and competence. I was getting quite annoyed with the whole fiasco by this stage and it was taking more and more self-control to prevent myself telling her that it wasn't my lack of skill that was the problem, it was her lack of calm and composure, and that if it wasn't for the animal then I would have told her to leave by now.

Once he was sedated, it was easier because he was less distressed, which calmed his owner down, and I managed to find a vein and he went peacefully off. Even then Mrs Young was far from grateful or apologetic, she still kept on about the fact that he'd suffered and wasn't it terrible that his last minutes were so awful, and that it had been so upsetting for her.

Clients like her are a vet's nightmare. Whatever I'd done would have been wrong, and everything was entirely my fault in her view. If she'd trusted me to do my best, then her dog wouldn't have suffered nearly as much as it did. It was always going to be a hard euthanasia to do quickly and completely stress-free due to the type of dog and its excitable nature, but if she'd just accepted that he might yelp as the needle went in and that he might struggle a bit, things would have been so much better. It really annoyed me that she didn't accept I was suitably qualified and demanded a more experienced vet. It would have made no difference which vet had been doing this, the result would have been the same, thanks to her. After five years at vet school and six months in practice, I consider myself to be qualified enough and skilful enough to perform routine tasks like this as well as any vet. I know she was upset and distressed, but so are most clients when their animals are put to sleep, and they don't react like that. They correctly assume you will do your best, and your best should be as good as any vet.

I told Emma about it when I got home last night and she was very supportive and said the woman had been entirely in the wrong. I was glad she was there to talk to so I could get it out of my system. It's really good at times like these to be seeing someone who's also a vet. Anyone else might have been sympathetic and supportive, but unless they'd been in similar situations, which most vets have been, they couldn't really understand or give a proper opinion on what I'd done.

Friday 16 May

Quiet at work. No more horrible clients thankfully, and no complaint from Mrs Young about Wednesday night. I almost wouldn't have minded if she had complained because then I could have really told her what I thought and defended myself against her unfair treatment. Anyway, let's just hope that there aren't too many more Mrs Youngs out there with ill and elderly pets, I don't think I could face a repeat performance.

Off for the weekend. Andy, an old school friend from home, is coming up this evening, which will be excellent. I haven't seen him for ages so it'll be good to catch up and hear what he's been up to in lovely Northamptonshire. Hopefully Hannah and some others are coming up tomorrow as well, so it should be a good weekend.

Monday 19 May

On Friday, Andy, Emma and I all went out for a relatively quiet night in Bideford. It was really good to see him again. He left school when we were sixteen and went to work for a boat-building company near where we grew up, so we haven't seen that much of each other in the last eight or nine years. Every time I go back home, though, we usually meet up, so we've kept in touch. It's strange how your friends change over the years. I was thinking about this the other day, all about how when I left university my circle of friends got much smaller but better, and it's the same when you leave school. While you are there you have a big group of friends, but when you leave you tend to keep in touch only with the people you really liked. Then you move on to college or a job and meet a new group of people, and the same happens when you leave, you select the friends who are true friends and stay in touch.

Anyway, on Saturday, Hannah, Tim, Nikkianna, Toby and Louise came down and, after spending the day on the beach and in the pub, we headed off into town to find a pub to get some food in. We eventually found a really nice place and had a good meal, then we noticed that there was karaoke about to start so we thought it might be worth staying for (we were pretty pissed by this point). We all had a few goes, but then something terrible happened – Hannah, Nik and Emma got up to sing something, and halfway through the DJ collapsed! At first we all thought he was messing around, but when an ambulance arrived a few minutes later and he was carried out, not moving, on a stretcher, we started to worry. No one seemed to know what had happened and we never did find out whether he lived or died, but it said something about the standard of our singing if we managed to kill the DJ with a rendition of 'Bohemian Rhapsody'! I hope he was OK.

After our murderous singing, we wandered back through town, stopping at a few more pubs, and ended up on the beach. It was a lovely mild spring evening so, as we were completely pissed, we all ended up swimming in the sea at half-past one in the morning.

It was great fun, splashing around; the water was lovely and warm, and it was really light and starry. It was one of those special nights that I'll remember for ages, no worrying about stroppy clients and ill animals, just messing around in the sea in the middle of the night with a group of friends. What more could you ask for?

I felt a little bit worried in the morning in case I'd done anything too embarrassing because I'm always aware that anyone in the town and the pubs could be one of our clients. The last thing that's going to instil confidence and respect into local animal lovers is seeing their vet cavorting around the town with a traffic cone on his head! (Not that I'd do anything like that of course!) It is a bit of a restriction, though, but I suppose you can't have it all. If you want to be respected and thought of as a good, professional vet then you can't really go around acting like a drunken student.

Tuesday 20 May

5.00 p.m. Good morning surgery today, because Ian and Keith had to do it! I was called out to a calving at Lake's which was quite tricky but went OK. The calf was alive and a heifer as well so the farmer was pleased. Dairy farmers tend to put about half of their cows to dairy-type bulls and half to beef-type, in the hope that about 25 per cent of calves will be female dairy-type to act as replacements for the old cows in the herd. Dairy-type bulls carry genes for high milk quality and yield in their female offspring, whereas beef-type bulls have a genetic make-up giving characteristics suitable for beef production, such as large, fast-growing muscles. The different requirements of animals bred for milk production or beef means that an animal bred for one purpose will not usually be suitable for the other. The beef-type calves are reared on the farm or sold to be reared elsewhere and provide valuable additional income, but the male dairy-type calves are much less valuable to the farmer because they don't have the right conformation to rear for beef, and obviously they can't replace the old milking cows. They used to be either killed, or reared for veal. Now that raising calves for veal has been banned in this country the calves are either still killed or sent abroad to be raised as veal. In a way, although it was obviously right to ban veal production in this country, it hasn't helped the welfare of the calves, because instead of being raised in a cruel way in this country, they are put through a long road and sea journey before being raised in a cruel way in another country.

Veal production is one of the worst instances of man putting animals through unnecessary suffering. The calves are reared in tiny pens where they can't turn around, and fed milk and minimal roughage. This is done so that their muscle is anaemic and pale, but causes terrible suffering in the calves, and all because people want to eat meat which is a particular colour. There are systems of producing similar-tasting calf meat which are much less cruel, but the meat is not as pale (because the calves are fed a suitable diet and are allowed to move around), and no one will buy it. I think this is a really bad example of humans taking advantage of animals and putting fancy restaurant traditions before basic animal welfare. People need to think about what they eat and not just follow the crowd and go along with what people have always taken as acceptable. I'm not saying that everyone should become a vegetarian, just that if we are going to use animals to provide food, we should try and make every effort to do it in the most humane way possible.

I sometimes think I should do more than just fill my diary with rantings and ravings about things like this, which I feel strongly about, and actually get out and do something positive like join one of the societies that campaign against animal cruelty. Maybe I will. I'll talk to Emma about it because she feels the same as me about these things.

Wednesday 21 May

2.35 p.m. Very bad mood! I've had one of those frustrating mornings when everything goes wrong. I was in a bad mood anyway because Blackie, the devil cat, got himself trapped in the spare room overnight, and in protest he left a nice pile of devil faeces on the spare bed. As a result, I was late in for morning surgery, which was packed of course, so I didn't finish until half past ten. Then I had what looked like a couple of fairly easy farm calls, one to do some routine scanning and fertility work, and the other to see some ill calves, but they turned out to be a disaster. Firstly I got confused between two farmers with the same surname (they're cousins I think) and ended up going miles to the wrong farm. When I finally got to the right farm, I had a twenty-minute discussion with the farmer about the other farmer's calves! I was wondering why he looked so confused while I was asking him about the coughing calves that I'd seen last week.

Anyway, after driving halfway across Devon and muddling up farmers and animals all morning, the last straw came when I was on the way home, looking forward to lunch, when Sue rang from the practice and told me that there was a calving back out at Brian Hill's.

The calving was one of the worst I've ever had to do. The calf had been dead for some time, and was rotten and very, very smelly. All the fluids from the womb had evaporated so it was all really dry and nasty. After putting in lots and lots of lubricant and manoeuvring the calf for twenty minutes, I eventually managed to ease it out. I was now not only in a foul mood but I smelt suitably foul as well. Usually most farms have a few stillbirths every year because there are so many common infections which can occasionally cause it. However, real problems can arise when a specific nasty infection like salmonella gets on to a farm and I suspect this is the problem here. It can sweep through a herd, causing not only lots of stillbirths, but also abortions, fertility problems and other illnesses such as diarrhoea.

I've just had a very thorough wash!

6.15 p.m. I talked to Ian about the calving when I got back to the surgery this afternoon, and he said they'd had quite a few cases of salmonella out at Brian Hill's farm, so he wouldn't be suprised if this turned out to be another one. He also said that he had his own method of diagnosing salmonella: he didn't waste the farmer's money on blood tests or faeces samples, he just looked at his arms in the few days after a suspect calving. If he came up in a rash, he could say pretty certainly that the cow had salmonella.

I'll keep an eye on my arms and see what happens!

Thursday 22 May

This is a summary of my working day today – consulting, neutering, consulting.

I think I'm beginning to realize that, although being a vet can be exciting and really rewarding, it's also a job like any other and can get pretty monotonous and dull after a while. Every morning I have to do an hour of morning surgery, which can be OK if there are some interesting cases in, or nice clients, but usually it gets quite tedious and repetitive. I enjoy surgery more, as it's a bit more challenging, and you don't have the pressure of having to be nice and polite to people all the time. It can get pretty stressful though if things start to go wrong. Farm work can also get a bit dull, especially if you're just doing routine pregnancy diagnoses or fertility checks, but I don't mind it as much because you get to go out and drive around and see the countryside, as opposed to being stuck inside all the time.

I sometimes wonder whether I'll still be a full-time vet in ten or twenty years' time. I'm certainly not sure that I can see myself getting to sixty-five and still be expressing anal glands and clipping rabbits' teeth. I suppose once you become a partner in a practice then the business side of things comes into your life and adds a bit more variety (and stress). Hopefully, what'll happen is that the grassboard or my book will be a massive success and make me rich, so I can just be a part-time vet. I think if you didn't have to do it day in, day out, it would be much more enjoyable.

I can dream I suppose!

Sunday 25 May

7.00 p.m. On call all weekend. Friday was quiet so I got a bit more book writing done (it's the first day of Ben's job and he's met nice old Mr Norton, who's taking him out on his first farm call), and took the grassboard out for some more trials (going very well, did my first 180° spin jump, which was excellent – if that's possible on an early prototype, just imagine what decent snowboarders will be able to do on the finished thing).

Saturday was quiet until the evening, when I got called out to what turned out to be a cow caesarean. I'd only done one before, so I was quite pleased to get another one to do on my own. The first one I did was soon after I qualified and Emma came and helped because she was over that night. It all went OK, but I think our relationship suffered more than the cow, because I was quite stressed and ended up ordering Emma around a bit, which she didn't take too kindly to!

Cow caesars seem to be a bit of a milestone in large-animal work. Once you've got a couple under your belt you get much more confidence in general, knowing that you can tackle a serious bit of large-animal surgery. It's been a contest amongst all our friends who are doing large-animal work to be the first to do a solo cow caesar, especially the blokes. In the end, I think it was Emma who did the first one, and has gone on to do quite a few, much to the frustration of Pat, who is very keen on large-animal work and has yet to have a go at one on his own.

This one went very smoothly, mainly due to the excellent facilities and helpful farmer rather than any great skill on my part. Some farmers expect you to try and perform a major abdominal operation in a dimly lit, muck-filled shed with nowhere to put your instruments and only half a bucket of cold muddy water to scrub-up in. This place was really good though. The cow was in a lovely, light barn, with a couple of bales acting as a table for the operating kit. The farmer's wife not only brought two steaming buckets of clean hot water, but also large mugs of hot tea for me and the farmer.

The operation is quite a straightforward procedure really, it's just the thought of making a big hole in the side of a cow and pulling out the calf, while she stands there oblivious to it all, that makes it daunting when you first attempt it. It's done under local anaesthetic of course, but even so it really amazes me how quietly the cow stands while you're up to your elbows in a hole in the side of the abdomen!

The farmer helped by pulling the calf out once I'd made the hole in the womb and got its two back legs up, and didn't seem at all bothered by the blood and gore. I think most farmers are pretty used to sad things and it doesn't affect them too much, but you still get the occasional one who turns a funny colour and has to rush off and fix a tractor or attend to an emergency fence repair or something.

Anyway, it all went well and the cow was looking good at the end of the op, licking her calf and generally acting as if nothing had happened. I wonder if they think, 'Bloody hell! Where did this great calf come from? I thought having a calf was supposed to be painful. That was easy!'

Today I went back to check on her, and she and the calf are both looking fine. The calf is really big, which was the main reason it wouldn't come out the normal way, so the farmer is thinking about keeping him as a bull. That gives him a better outlook for life than most male calves, he'll get to live to a (relatively) ripe old age spending his days servicing herds of cows. A bit better than an exhausting twenty-four-hour lorry journey and then four months in a tiny pen being fed milk.

Monday 26 May

Rash! It's been coming on since Friday, but this morning when I woke up both my forearms were covered in little red pimples so I think that cow must have salmonella. I sent some samples off to the lab to confirm it because I wasn't convinced by Ian's theory and the results should be back by the end of the week, so I'll be able to see if my arms are an accurate salmonella detector or not.

I wrote some more book last night. It's getting hard to keep the momentum going now; I'm a bit bogged down. Maybe I need to get things going with the first hints that all is not as it seems in sunny Raunton. This is the latest bit that I did last night, where Ben's out on his first solo farm call.

> Ben made his way to the farm with the map unfolded on his lap, alternating between looking out for oncoming cars and trying to navigate his way through the maze of small country lanes. After several wrong turns and a small dent in the front of the practice car, he arrived at South View farm, which was one of the largest dairy farms on the practice books. It lay nestled at the foot of the moor, and was approached via a long winding lane. Ben was nervous as he drove up towards the farm buildings, thinking through what he was planning to do with the sick cow he was going to see.
>
> 'Cow with bad mastitis out at Young's,' Harry Norton had said. 'That'll be a good 'un for you to

start off with. I'm sure you'll be OK. Just remember what you learnt at college and you'll be fine.'

Suddenly Ben was jolted from his thoughts as he heard a small bang, and felt the car bump as if it had gone over a large rock. Looking back he could see the motionless shape of a pheasant lying on the road.

'Bugger!' he exclaimed under his breath. This was not the perfect start to his first farm call.

I think a few true-life experiences will give the book a more realistic feel. Hopefully, I'll get past this little bit of writer's block, because I'd really like to finish it and writing a book is something I've always wanted to do.

Tuesday 27 May

8.15 a.m. Emma came over last night, and she's taken Pan and Badger off with her today because they're going to be castrated. I couldn't face doing it so Emma's going to do them both.

I was reluctant to have them done at first, I suppose it's typical male-sympathy behaviour. Emma was very keen, because she's a strong believer that all pets should be neutered both to try and reduce the number of unwanted animals around, and because of the health benefits to the animals. She is right, it's best for them, but part of me still feels that it's not fair to deprive them of their doghood. There's no logic in feeling how I do, I know they'll be happier and healthier without them, but still there is a little part of me that wants to let them grow into full male dogs. Thinking rationally, depriving them of their bits is a small price to pay for the health benefits – no prostate cancer, no prostatitis, no testicular cancer. They'd thank us if they knew!

I hope they make it through the operation OK, I'd be so upset if anything happened to either of them. I trust Emma as much as any vet, if not more, so I'm not really worried . . .

but you never know what could go wrong. Bonnie's owners probably thought that nothing would go wrong and look what happened to her.

11.50 a.m. Emma's just rung and they're both round from their anaesthetics and looking fine. I'm so relieved! Apparently Badger was a real wimp and had to be held down by three people before Emma could give him the anaesthetic injection. I hope he doesn't bear a grudge.

7.00 p.m. They're back in one piece (although slightly lighter!). They both walked in and immediately went to sleep; they looked exhausted. I hope they don't suffer from any nasty post-op complications like poor old Toby – I'd hate to see them suffer like he did. Also there's no way I want to spend a week sleeping on the kitchen floor.

Wednesday 28 May

Pan and Badger doing very well. Emma has given me Pan's bits preserved in formalin to have as a memento. I'm not sure what to do with them really, I don't think they'd go too well on the mantelpiece alongside the ornaments.

Thursday 29 May

Pan and Badger still doing very well. I had a look at the wounds and although I don't like to admit it, Emma's made a very neat job of the operations. She's always been really keen on surgery, and I think she's getting quite good at it. (I'd never tell her that of course!)

The main problem she's got at the moment is that her practice is mainly large-animal and the small-animal operating facilities are basic to say the least. Some places, like Toby's practice, have brand new anaesthetic machines, state of the art respiratory monitors, completely sterile operating theatres and a full team of qualified nurses, whereas small country practices such as Emma's tend to make do with old equipment, clean rather than sterile operating theatres and, often, untrained nurses. Standards may be lower and levels of post-operative problems are higher. It also restricts what operations can be safely attempted, it's no use trying complex orthopaedic operations if you can't ensure that everything is sterile because the risks of post-op infection are too high.

I think Emma finds this a bit restricting and I can see she's probably going to want to move on to a better equipped, more small-animal-oriented practice before long.

I'm pretty lucky in Bideford, because although it's not a high-powered, ultra-modern small-animal practice, it is quite up to date and is much better than a lot of practices.

Friday 30 May

Lab results came back for the cow from Brian Hill's farm and, guess what, they're positive for salmonella. It looks as though my arms are as sensitive as Ian's. Next time I'll trust the old ways rather than resorting to these new-fangled laboratory tests.

Saturday 31 May

On call last night, and I had to go and see a vomiting dog at 10 p.m. It was just a mild case of gastroenteritis so I hope it'll respond to the injections I gave. No mention of plastic bags, so it doesn't look like being a second Jake Johnson!

Did morning surgery with Ian, who's on for the weekend, and now I'm off until Monday. The only interesting thing this morning was seeing the dog that fell off the cliff a few weeks ago. The owner brought him in because he'd been in a fight with another dog. He was OK, nothing more than a small cut and some scratches. I think this dog is rapidly using up his supply of luck.

June

Sunday 1 June

Ben looked worried as Jasper vomited for the third time on the kitchen floor. This time there were specks of blood in the yellow liquid that was staining the towel on which the ill collie was lying.

'I think we're going to have to operate on him, Mrs Smith,' he said, standing up to face the elderly owner. 'There must be something stuck for him to still be vomiting like this after all the treatment he's had.'

'Yes, I think there must be,' she replied sadly. 'He's always chewing at things. I mean, as I said a few days ago, he was having a go at my husband's slippers last week before he got ill. You don't thing he could have swallowed them, do you?'

Ben paused, he'd constantly dismissed Mrs Smith's slipper theory throughout Jasper's illness, but now he was coming to realize that she may well have been right all along. The main thing was to get him well again, he told himself, not to worry about mistakes he may have made along the way.

'It's possible,' he finally admitted, 'but we won't know until we have a look.'

This is Ben's first night on duty alone and he'd been called out late at night to see Jasper, a dog who'd been vomiting over the last week. Ben finally decides to operate. But what will he find when he gets to the practice? I'm getting quite excited writing this, so hopefully that means it might be good to read.

I'm over my writer's block now and it's flowing well.

Ben carried Jasper to the car and carefully placed him on the back seat. 'Don't worry, Mrs Smith, I'll do everything I can. I'm sure he's going to be fine,' he said as he reversed the car on to the road, feeling much less confident than he sounded.

When he pulled up outside the practice he was surprised to see Peter's car standing in the car park. Ben breathed a sigh of relief, at least he would have some help if Peter was around. He hadn't been looking forward to trying to perform the major surgery that Jasper needed on his own, so soon after qualifying. Ben had found Peter quite difficult to fathom: sometimes he was fairly friendly, but most of the time he seemed cold and reserved. Maybe working together as a team on this case would help to break the ice a little, thought Ben as he unlocked the surgery door and carried the collapsed dog through towards the theatre.

Monday 2 June

1.15 p.m. Went to take the stitches out of the cow caesar after morning surgery today. It was looking really good, the wound had healed nicely and the cow was eating and generally behaving as if nothing had happened. I was very relieved that it had gone so well, because although it's really quite a simple operation, it's still something that can easily go wrong. I've heard quite a few horror stories from friends who have seen vets make a real mess of the operation, or where the cow has collapsed mid-op and rolled over on to the open wound!

The BBC are coming down again this week to do some more filming. I'm really starting to look forward to having them around. I think it's because I've got used to being filmed, so I don't get too worried any more, and also I'm getting to know the crews and directors fairly well. Most of the camera- and soundmen are really nice and have some excellent stories to tell about places they've been to and people they've filmed.

One of the cameramen told me last time they were down about filming with Michael Palin on his Pacific rim adventure series, which sounded so exciting. I think I might re-train as a cameraman, it sounds much better than being a vet!

Tuesday 3 June

I had to rush out to see a calf this morning as soon as I got to work. The farmer rang up and said that one of his year-lings was bloated up, so I left a full waiting room of people for Ian and Keith and headed straight out to the farm, near Hartland.

This is one of our decent dairy farms and instead of sending their beef calves off to be reared elsewhere, they have their own separate unit for calf rearing. It was one of these fattening calves that the farmer took me too when I arrived, and I could immediately see the problem – the calf's abdomen was bloated to nearly double its usual size and the calf was in a very bad state, collapsed on the floor of the pen.

Bloat like this can be rapidly life-threatening, so I rushed back to the car and fetched a stomach tube. With the farmer's help I passed the tube down towards the calf's forestomach, expecting a jet of gas and liquid to shoot out, relieving the bloat. However, I couldn't get the tube more than halfway down the calf's oesophagus, where it encountered some solid blockage.

'Have these calves been eating potatoes or anything?' I asked. One possibility was that the calf could have something like a piece of potato stuck in its throat.

'No, nothing like that, just grain and hay. I'm always very careful now because I had a couple die a few years back from getting potatoes stuck.'

The calf was starting to look worse and worse. 'I'm going to have to make a hole in the abdomen to let the gas out,' I said hurriedly, as I ran back to the car. I opened the boot and searched frantically for the plastic trochar designed to make a neat and fairly sterile hole in the animal's flank. As I rummaged around in my recently installed boot container, I remembered that yesterday I'd cleaned everything out and I must have left the box with all my surgical stuff at the practice.

No need to panic, I told myself, I'll use a scalpel blade, and then try and stitch the edges after I've got the calf sorted out. I rummaged again, and then the horrible realization came over me that all my scalpel blades were in the box with the trochar, back at the practice. Now I did panic! The calf was going to die unless I could relieve the bloat within the next few minutes, and I had left all the necessary instruments at the practice.

I was on the verge of desperation. The farmer was calling out that the calf was almost gone when, at last, I spotted a knife in the bottom of one of the compartments of the boot-box. It was an unused knife that had been given to me a few weeks earlier by a drugs rep. I grabbed it and rushed back to the calf, which was looking pretty unsavable. I considered trying to make the site where I was going to operate a little more sterile, but I thought the calf would be dead by the time I'd gone back to the car and fetched some disinfectant, so I just cleaned off the worst of the muck with my hand. I looked at the recumbent, unmoving calf and worked out the correct place to make a hole to relieve the bloat. There was no time for any anaesthetic but the animal was unconscious by this point, so I took the knife and plunged it into his flank. Once the knife was through into the stomach I twisted it to open up the hole, and immediately a jet of gas and liquid shot out.

The calf didn't move. I looked at its eyes and felt for a heartbeat, and sank back into the straw – it was dead.

'Too late I'm afraid,' I told the farmer, who was leaning on the gate, looking resigned at the loss of a valuable animal.

It would have almost certainly died even if I'd had the proper stuff with me. After they've been bloated for some time they get poisoned by the build-up of acid in the blood, and you have to get to them pretty quickly to be able to correct this before they get to the collapsed state in which this one was.

Still, I felt quite bad that I'd had to resort to such a basic and primitive technique to try and save the calf. I should have made sure I had the proper instrument with me before I set off. The farmer is probably off telling all the other farmers in the area how the vet came out to see an ill calf and ended up stabbing it with a 'Leo Animal Health' pocket knife, and surprisingly it didn't survive!

When I got back to the practice I made sure that I put the instrument box back in the car – I don't ever want to have to go through the panic I went through this morning again. I suppose in a way I was very lucky to have had the pocket knife, because if I hadn't had that I would have been completely stuffed. Although the calf died, at least the farmer saw me try my best to save it. If I'd just turned around and said, 'I'm sorry, I've forgotten the instrument box so there's nothing I can do,' he would have been a lot more upset, even though the end result would have been the same.

I'm just glad that the BBC aren't coming until tomorrow. This would have been an excellent exciting case for them, but not something I'd really have wanted broadcast.

Friday 6 June

BBC are still here. They've been really lucky the last few days because they've had some excellent stories.

They turned up on Wednesday, and the first case they filmed turned out to be pretty interesting. It was a dog with a really painful mass on one side of the base of its tail. I told the owner, Mr Norman, that I thought it was either an abscess or a nasty tumour but, because it was so painful, we'd have to sedate him to have a proper look. Like many others he was quite upset when I mentioned the word tumour, so I really hoped that when we had sedated him it would turn out to be an abscess or something else treatable.

Some owners get quite confused by the terms 'tumour' and 'neoplasia' (both terms are used to describe cancer), and there have been a few instances where I've said to people that their animal has a tumour and they've replied, 'Oh, that's good, isn't it? At least he hasn't got cancer.' I think that people are much more scared by the word 'cancer' and immediately associate it with nasty invasive growths which kill very quickly, whereas terms like 'tumour' or 'malignant neoplasm' are less well understood and people don't necessarily think of them as such serious problems.

Anyway, we sedated Ricky and I was able to examine the mass more closely. After a couple of minutes I was still unsure exactly what was going on because although from the outside the mass felt solid and very much like a tumour, when I felt inside his back end with a finger, I could feel lots of small stones in the area where the mass was. I asked Ian to come and have a feel and after a couple of minutes he made a diagnosis.

'It's, er, a perennial hernia,' he said, 'full of stones.'

The cameras were filming all the action and after making his diagnosis, Ian left as rapidly as possible. I don't think he minds the cameras too much, but he avoids them when at all possible. He's really good when he is filmed, because he's full of stories about how it was being a vet when he qualified and has lots of amusing anecdotes about vets and clients. He comes over as very natural – I think he just doesn't really care what the public think. The crew always says that these are the people who come across the best because they are relaxed, and the people who look silly and are disliked by the public are those who try to make a real effort to be funny or look good. I hope I come across OK when the series comes out. It's going to be really strange when it does, I wonder if Emma and me will get recognized in the street and things.

I'm looking forward to it, but it's going to be very odd seeing our ugly mugs on BBC1 knowing that ten million people are watching!

As soon as Ian said perennial hernia, I thought, Of course! Why didn't I think of that? It's one of those cases where as soon as someone else solves it, it becomes so obvious that you can't believe you failed to see it yourself. A perennial hernia is where the muscles surrounding the back end become weak and a pouch of back passage can form which pushes out under the skin to form a swelling to one side of the tail. The pouch then tends to fill up with faeces, which become hard and painful, as it had in Ricky's case.

Once the problem was clear, I could start to empty the hernia using a gloved finger. It was one of the worst, most disgusting jobs I've yet had to do as a vet. The hernia was impacted with a mix of stones and faeces and the smell was horrific, even through a face mask. It took about twenty minutes to clear it all out, and by the end the camera crew were looking distinctly green, and even Helen, an experienced nurse who'd smelt more foul smells in her time than most, was finding the stench almost unbearable!

It was worth the effort, though, because once Ricky came round from the sedative, he immediately looked so much happier and relieved. He ran back into the waiting room to his owner and jumped up wagging his tail as if to say, 'Thank you, master, thank you.'

Mr Norman was overjoyed when I explained what we'd found and told him that the outlook was good as long as he could stop Ricky from eating any more stones. However, I did warn him that if the swelling came back we may have to think about operating on it to repair the hernia permanently.

'Thank God it wasn't cancer. I was so worried,' said Mr Norman, rubbing Ricky's tummy. 'He's been such a great dog, so loyal and faithful, I just couldn't bear it if anything happened to him.'

It was a really good story for the BBC, and a good case

for me as well because I felt as though I'd really done some good and helped an animal. Ricky had come in in agony and gone home happy and well.

On Thursday I took Badger's and Pan's stitches out. The wounds had healed up beautifully. The BBC had filmed Emma when she did the castration, so they filmed the stitches coming out to complete the story.

Over the last few days it's really amused me the way the clients act with the BBC around. Once they know the cameras are going to be there they become either shy and reluctant to come in at all, or go the other way and bring their animals in for trivial problems which they'd normally not bother with, just so they can get on TV. It's really funny to see the middle-aged ladies in the waiting room dressed up in their best clothes, hair immaculately coiffed, made up to the nines, with their little Yorkshire terriers and miniature poodles. They tend to be very disappointed when they bring their dog in for nail clipping or something else routine and the camera crew fail to appear because the case is not exciting enough.

The funniest ones tend to be the farmers. They are usually dressed in muck-covered ripped overalls, but when they hear that the cameras are on their way, they rush into the farm-house and put on a freshly washed and ironed shirt and pair of trousers. Ever since the first time the BBC came and I panicked about the state of my trousers, I've given up worrying what I look like when they're around. I think I may regret this once I see myself on TV in some of the bloodstained shirts and torn trousers that I've worn.

I'm off from this afternoon. Hopefully there'll be some surf, because I'm itching for a decent session, I haven't been in for ages.

Sunday 8 June

8.30 p.m. I'm in trouble! We were having an excellent weekend until this Saturday afternoon, when disaster struck. We decided to go surfing down at a place called Bantham on the south Devon coast as there wasn't any surf on the north coast, and Emma and I headed off after lunch. We met Toby at Exeter and he followed us down.

I borrowed Ian's car for the weekend because he's off in Austria (visiting royal relatives!) and my practice car is in the garage. It's a brand-new estate car in spotless condition so I was told to look after it and not get it muddy or scratched on pain of death. I didn't get it too muddy or scratched, but unfortunately I have completely bashed one front corner in!

We were about a mile from the sea, driving down a wet country lane, when a car came round a corner towards us. I slammed on the brakes but we just skidded on the muddy surface. The lane was too narrow to allow any manoeuvring, so we ended up smashing into the front of the other car (which had managed to stop). The impact wasn't too bad and we can't have been going too fast as the airbag didn't fire, but the damage was pretty nasty, the whole driver's side front corner was crumpled in. The only casualty was Pan, who was on the back seat and ended up wedged behind the passenger seat. He was unhurt though, and once we'd freed him he seemed pretty unfazed by the whole affair. The other car was fairly unscathed as it had bull bars to protect it, but the driver was still quite angry. We exchanged insurance details and after freeing the mangled bodywork from the wheel with a calving jack (very useful, every motorist should have one!) we managed to carry on and make it to the beach. I guess the theory that most newly qualified vets crash their car in their first year of practice has another supporting statistic.

The most annoying thing about the whole incident was that when we got to the sea, we found that instead of the clean four-foot swell predicted, there was one to two feet of onshore wind-blown waves, which were barely surfable. Crashing the boss's car for classic surf is almost worth it, whereas crashing the boss's car for some of the worst surf I've ever seen was definitely not worthwhile!

On Sunday, after going out in Bridgewater on Saturday night to drown our sorrows, we took the grassboard to the Quantox so that Toby and Tom could try it out. They both thought it was brilliant and by the end of a couple of hours were cruising down the hills really well. They survived relatively uninjured, and said they'll buy one when I get it into production. I think the next stage is going to be to finalize the design and look into mass production. I might need to borrow some money or find some investors, but I think it's definitely got a future.

11.00 p.m. Oh God! What is Ian going to say when he sees the mess I've made of his lovely new car?

1.15 a.m. Maybe I could lie and say that someone backed into me in a car park? Or perhaps he won't notice if I park it in the shadows?

2.05 a.m. I'll blame Pan – I'll say that he jumped on me and made me crash.

2.15 a.m. No, it's no good, I'm going to have to admit what happened and take the blame. What's the worst thing that can happen anyway . . . ?

Monday 9 June

8.30 a.m. . . . being sacked, having to pay for the damage, being resoundingly thrashed with a wet calving rope, the possibilities are endless!

10.30 a.m. Well, I'm still alive and I've still got a job, although the calving rope weals are still sore! Ian took it pretty well, really. I decided to get it over with as soon as I arrived so I walked in and told him that I had had a little accident in his car and he'd better come and have a look.

He didn't say much but came out and looked at the damage.

'Oh dear,' he said in a resigned tone. 'I suppose it was bound to happen sooner or later, but why did it have to be in my car?'

'I'm really sorry,' I said. 'It was the mud on the road, I just couldn't stop in time.'

He sorted out the insurance and booked the car into a garage for the repairs. As my penance, he's now got my car and I'm driving the garage courtesy car, which is a knackered old Ford Fiesta!

Tuesday 10 June

5.00 p.m. Had to see a horse today, which is always a bit of a novelty. We don't have many horse clients on the books, and most of the ones we do have Ian tends to see, so I don't really get to do very much equine work at all. This suits me fine because, although I like horses and find the work quite interesting, I feel very unsure about dealing with horsy owners. I don't mind going to see a horse that's owned by a farmer because he's likely to say, 'Ar, 'ee's lame on 'is back pin, and 'ee's a birt swollen down thur like.' Which translates easily to, 'He is lame in his back leg, which is swollen at the bottom.' Whereas if a horsy owner wanted to communicate the same point they would say something like, 'Oh yes, he's been favouring his nearside hind somewhat, and he's got a bog spavin coming on. Maybe also a touch of thoroughpin, wouldn't you say?'

I get a bit intimidated by all the strange words and then assume that the owner is much more knowledgeable about horses than I am. If I could just ignore that intimidation and look at the horse like any other animal, I'm sure I'd be fine.

I suppose it's a matter of confidence as well; as I haven't seen many horses since I qualified I feel much less confident about remembering all the stuff we learnt at college relating to them, whereas with cows and small animals, which I treat every day, I'm constantly using and refreshing my knowledge.

Anyway, this horse was owned by a nice, non-horsy, owner called Miss Roberts, who lives near the practice. The horse was an elderly ex-hunter called Eric, and he'd had diarrhoea for a few days. I checked him over and he didn't look too bad so I gave her some worming paste to give him, as he hadn't been wormed for some time, and put him on some antibiotic powders.

That should sort him out, and then I can say that I actually cured a horse!

Wednesday 11 June

8.55 a.m. Bloody crap Fiesta won't start.

9.10 a.m. Finally made it to work. Jamie, one of the nurses, had to come and pick me up in her battered old Metro van that usually carries her pack of slobbering St Bernards around. The Fiesta is being picked up by the garage and thankfully Ian's car should be ready by this afternoon, so I can get mine back again.

6.45 p.m. Just finished evening surgery, which was pretty quiet. I did get my car back today, which was a relief. That Fiesta was a death trap!

On call this evening.

11.45 p.m. I really can't believe some people. I got called out at half-past ten to see a dog which had been hit by a car, and the bloke has just had a real go at me about the fact that it's cost him £60. What does he expect? That we'll come out at his beck and call free of charge?

It really annoys me the way people complain about out-

Right: Emma
and me on our
Graduation Day

Below: Pan keeps
a watchful eye on
lambing proceedings

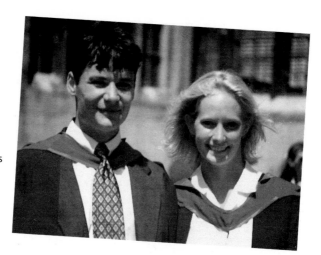

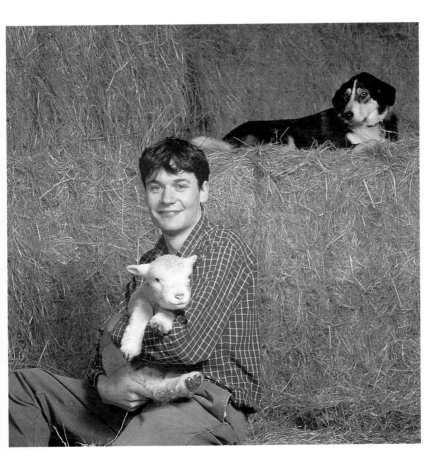

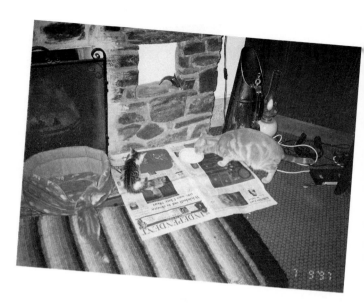

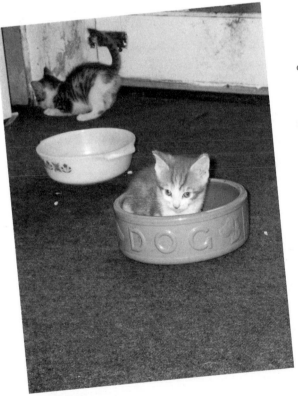

Above: Charlie the cat with new kittens, Nigel and Brian

Left: The kittens make a dog's dinner of their first day

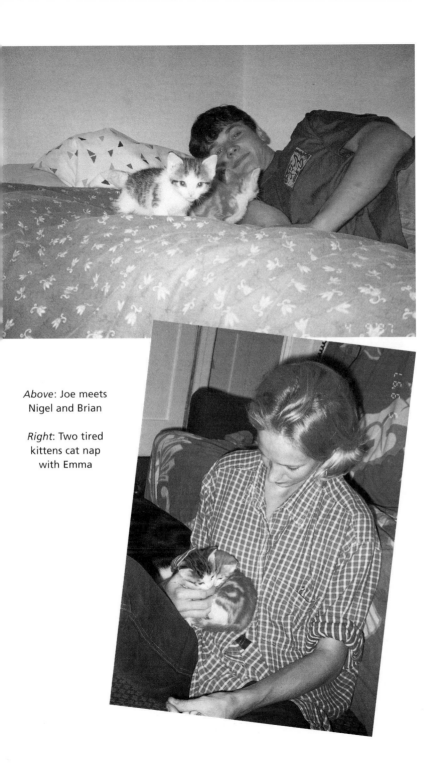

Above: Joe meets
Nigel and Brian

Right: Two tired
kittens cat nap
with Emma

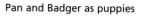

Pan and Badger as puppies

Right: It's my bed Badger!

Below: Oh alright we'll
share it then!

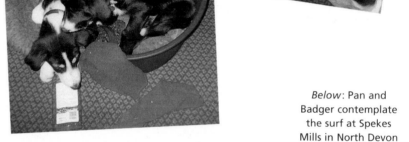

Below: Pan and
Badger contemplate
the surf at Spekes
Mills in North Devon

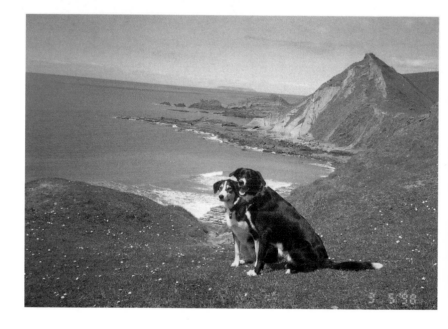

The start of a
drunken weekend

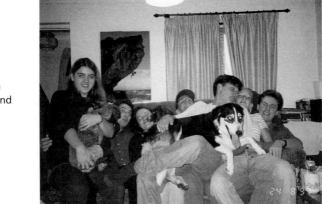

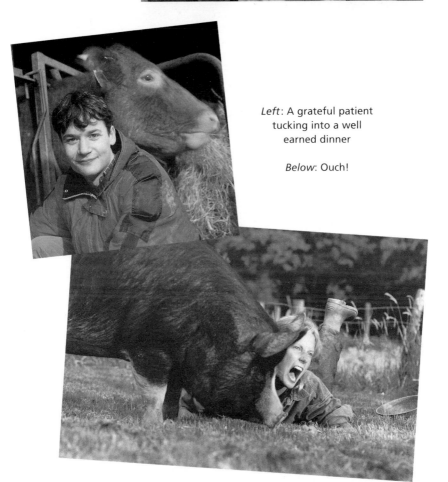

Left: A grateful patient
tucking into a well
earned dinner

Below: Ouch!

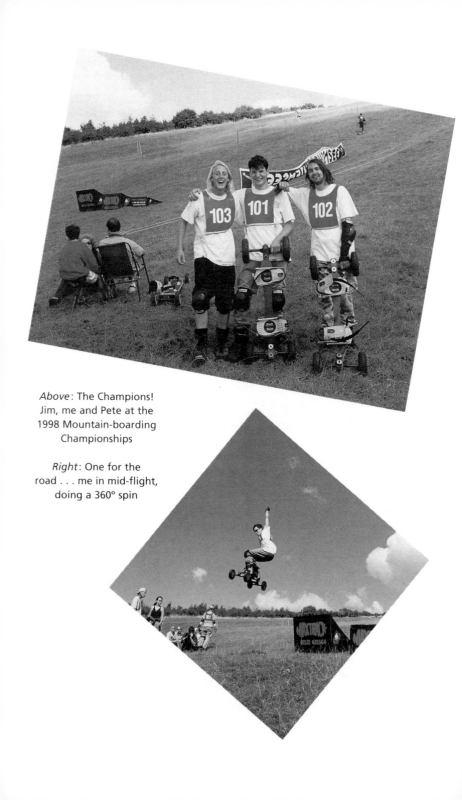

Above: The Champions!
Jim, me and Pete at the
1998 Mountain-boarding
Championships

Right: One for the
road . . . me in mid-flight,
doing a 360° spin

Just married!
Outside the
registry office

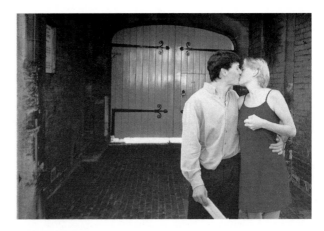

Left: The speeches,
complete with 'Vets in
Practice' film crew

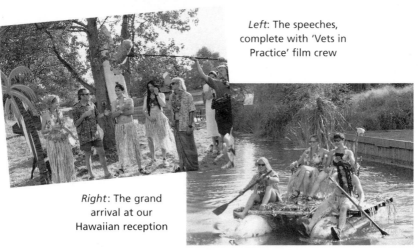

Right: The grand
arrival at our
Hawaiian reception

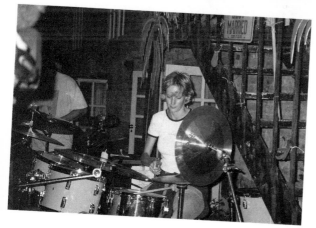

Left: Emma
drumming with
The Babysitters

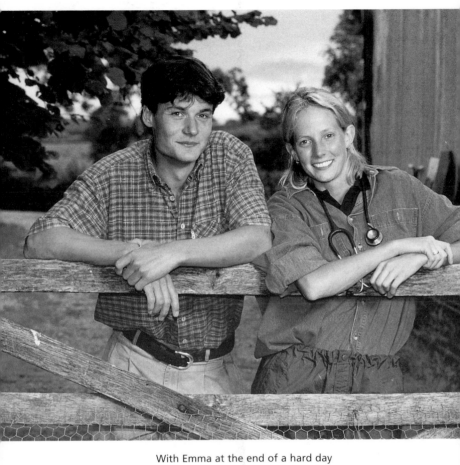

With Emma at the end of a hard day

of-hours charges. I don't think that charging £60 to see an emergency case, check it over and give it some treatment at eleven at night is at all unreasonable. I told this bloke he should try and get a plumber to come out and fix a leaking pipe at eleven at night for £60 and see what response he gets. It's the same old problem, though, people assume that because it's an animal, it's different. I know being a vet isn't like other jobs and a love of animals and caring for them at all times are essential parts of the job, but it is, at the same time, a way of earning a living and people seem to forget that. They should think about the possibility of their animal needing emergency veterinary treatment in the middle of the night and be prepared to pay for it. If they can't afford to look after their animals then they're not in a position to own one.

I'm not saying that if you haven't got lots of money you shouldn't keep pets, it's just that many people seem to think it's their absolute right to have pets even if they can't really afford them. It's not fair on the animals if you're not going to be able to look after them if they need help. All vets are obliged to look after all the animals in their care and will never refuse to treat a truly ill animal, and I think some people tend to take advantage of this fact. They know the vet won't refuse to help and they'll get treatment for their animal, even if they have no intention of paying for it.

Maybe the solution is either a national NHS-type service where all animal owners pay an annual tax and then get free treatment at certain special practices, or perhaps all animal owners should be obliged to take out some form of pet insurance. I know nothing like this is likely ever to happen, so vets will continue to be taken advantage of in order that people's pets are properly looked after.

Thursday 12 June

7.00 p.m. Boring day today. Managed to get a bit of writing done between surgeries this afternoon. I'm really getting into the swing of it now, it seems almost to be writing itself. I'm sure when I look back and read it I'll realize what utter rubbish it is, but I'm enjoying doing it so I think it's worth carrying on.

The plot's developing quite nicely. Ben almost caught Peter red-handed (literally) when he took Jasper through to the operating theatre late at night to remove the slipper from his intestines. Luckily for Peter (and the plot), he had just finished his evil surgery and was able to get away without Ben finding out what was going on. The seeds of suspicion are being sown, though, because the next morning Ben makes a strange discovery:

Ben arrived early in order to check on Jasper. The operation had taken until past midnight, and he had sat with the dog as he came round from his anaesthetic into the early hours of the morning. Jasper had been awake and looking pretty well when he'd left, but he was still feeling very nervous as he rushed through the front door of the practice and ran down to the kennels.

'Don't worry, he's fine,' said Emily, smiling at Ben's worried face. 'He's up and looking brilliant.'

Ben looked past the young nurse and saw that, as she said, Jasper was up in his kennel, wagging his long bushy tail, looking bright and obviously wondering what all the fuss was about.

'Thank God!' breathed Ben. Relief swept over him as he knelt down and stroked the collie's head. 'Thank you, Jasper,' he whispered. 'You're a fine dog.'

As he made a fuss of Jasper, a shiny object suddenly caught his eye through the open door. It was lying underneath the anaesthetic trolley in the operating theatre.

'There's those scissors we lost yesterday,' he

exclaimed to Emily, and walked over to retrieve them. However, instead of the scissors that Ben was expecting, he stood up holding a bloody surgical instrument.

'That's a weird clamp. I'm sure we didn't use that last night,' he said, bemused. 'Oh well, maybe it's been there for a while. Perhaps it's one of Peter's strange orthopaedic instruments or something. I'll ask him later on.'

As he turned to walk back to the office he put the mysterious object down on the table, but as he moved away he noticed something odd – the blood that was staining the instrument was now on his fingers.

The plot thickens!

Sunday 15 June

Quiet weekend on call (so far). On Friday I had a busy morning operating:

One bitch spay (nice easy Jack Russell, no problem!)
Two cat spays
One lump removal from leg of elderly spaniel (quite tricky but went OK)
One dental on a Yorkie (yuk)
Hamster leg amputation! (Had broken leg, which wasn't very fixable, so instead I removed the leg. It's running around the cage looking fine!)

On Saturday, morning surgery was average, and then I had a couple of farm calls to do. In the afternoon I want to the hunt kennels over at Torrington to have a look at the carcass of a cow which had died at Tony Fulford's farm. It was a bit grim, but really interesting to see the place. It's where we send all the cows which die or are so ill they can't be sent to the slaughterhouse because of meat hygiene regulations, and they end up as hunting-hound food. The place is on a big country estate, and the slaughter place is in an old outbuilding. They had just started butchering Mr Fulford's cow when I arrived, and as I watched they pulled the hide off with a mechanical winch.

I've seen slaughterhouses before. When we were at college we got shown round a few different ones, but it was still a bit horrible seeing a poor old cow being pulled apart like that. I'm used to putting them back together not taking them apart!

As soon as the hide was off I could see immediately what the cow had died of. All the fat under the skin was bright yellow instead of the normal white colour, which was a clear indication that the cow had been suffering from acute liver disease. When the liver doesn't work properly, bile and other metabolic by-products build up in the system and cause jaundice, which is what had happened to this cow.

Mr Fulford has had a few cows suffering from acute liver disease recently and it's almost definitely due to poor nutrition. Some of the information I got from that talk back in March will be useful in trying to help prevent any more cases.

Sunday has been really quiet so far, all I've had to do is see one cat that was hit by a car (no real damage; very lucky). It's been quite sunny so I took the grassboard out this afternoon. I made up a small wooden ramp and did a few jumps on it – it works really well. The flexibility of the board gives loads of 'boing' as you take off and land which means I was able to get pretty high and the landings weren't too painful!

I've just finished doing a bit more to the novel. I've introduced the love interest (Sarah, the new vet nurse) and sown a few more seeds of suspicion in Ben's mind about what Peter is up to:

Surprise flashed across Peter's normally passive face as Ben showed him the mysterious instrument found under the anaesthetic trolley.

'Ah, er, that's mine,' he said hurriedly, snatching it away from Ben. 'It's out of the orthopaedic kit. It must have fallen there last week when I operated on that German shepherd's leg.'

Ben didn't mention the fresh blood that was staining the instrument when he found it that morning.

Why was Peter being so secretive and obviously lying about when it'd been used? thought Ben as he drove off to his first farm call of the day. Perhaps he was operating on the side to earn some extra money without Mr Norton finding out?

As he was pondering the problem, Ben's eyes wandered from the road in front, but were suddenly jerked back into focus by the sight of a car coming rapidly towards him round the corner of the narrow country lane. He slammed on the brakes, but the muddy road held no grip for the tyres and the car skidded out of control towards the oncoming car.

Monday 16 June

12.45 p.m. Went back to see Eric, the horse with diarrhoea, this morning. He's gone downhill since I last saw him. Now he's just standing in his stable hanging his head low and looking thoroughly dejected. His temperature had gone up as well, so I think he could have something more serious than just mild diarrhoea.

I took a faeces sample and sent it off to the lab to check for things like salmonella. If it is salmonella, the outlook is pretty poor, especially in a relatively old horse like him. I hope it comes back as negative because he's a lovely horse, and his owners are nice too.

7.00 p.m. Ricky, the dog with the bottom full of stones, came to evening surgery tonight. He's looking fine, so much better than he was before we cleared his problem. Mr Norman was very happy and relieved to see Ricky back to his old self again. He told me that when he was younger, Ricky used to regularly get on the bus from Northam to Westward Ho! on his own and go for a round trip into town and back. He also knew lots of different objects by name to fetch, such as 'fetch the slippers' or 'fetch the paper'. I really love dogs like Ricky, he's friendly, clever, loyal and a really good companion to his master. This is how all dogs should be, rather than being bred for their looks and appearance and exploited by their owners, who only want them to win them prizes in shows and to show off with. Keeping a pet is about providing an animal with a good home in return for companionship and affection, and shouldn't be about treating animals as toys or status symbols. Animal breeding and showing is, in my opinion, exploitation of animals, and is responsible for an awful lot of unnecessary animal suffering.

Tuesday 17 June

Bad news. Eric has come back positive for salmonella. I told Miss Roberts and explained that although the outlook was pretty bad, it would be worth trying to treat him as there is a chance that he'll pull through.

I've changed the antibiotic to a stronger one which is very effective against salmonella, and told her to feed him hay and fresh grass rather than any feed concentrate. I also warned Miss Roberts about the risks from the bacteria, as salmonella can cause nasty infections in people. She seemed to feel it was worth taking the risk if it meant giving the horse a chance.

I really don't think his chances are much better than 50:50, but I'm going to keep my fingers crossed and see what happens. Animals can always surprise you.

Friday 20 June

Not a good few days. I've been getting really annoyed with having to take morning surgery every day. There's supposed to be a rota for doing the different surgeries and operating, but Ian and Keith don't ever stick to it, so I end up doing most of everything. Today, for example, Keith was supposed to be doing morning surgery but, as usual, he sat around fiddling with the computer, ignoring the rapidly filling waiting room. In the end I had no choice but to get on and start consulting; if I hadn't, the clients could have been waiting hours for Keith finally to give in and see them.

I'm also getting a little bit bored with some of the work. A lot of it is getting slightly repetitive and dull, especially the small-animal stuff. We don't seem to get that many really exciting cases in; all I end up doing most of the time is routine vaccinations and things. I suppose every now and then we get interesting cases, like Jake Johnson and Ricky, but they seem few and far between.

I started looking through the *Veterinary Record* job section this morning. I'm not really thinking of moving, but I suppose if I saw something particularly good advertised I might have to have a serious think about how long I want to stay here.

I like all the people here, especially Ian, who has been a great boss to have for my first job, and I also like the area. The main things I don't like, apart from some aspects of the job, are the fact that we're so far from all our friends, and that there isn't an awful lot to do here apart from surf (which can be great, but most of the time it's either flat or there's a howling gale). The nearest decent cinema is in Taunton, which is about an hour and a half away!

Also, being so far apart isn't good for me and Emma. We do see each other a lot, but we tend to be really knackered because of having to drive forty miles after work, and then get up really early to drive back in the morning. We have thought about Emma trying to get a job in Bideford or Barnstaple so that we could live together, but I think she would prefer to move back somewhere nearer our friends and a bit of civilization. Dulverton is even worse than Bideford in terms of being cut off from the outside world. It's such a small town that everyone knows everyone else's business. When Emma first turned up to start her job last year, she pulled up in her car having never been there except for her interview and, as soon as she started unloading her stuff, an old woman came up to her and said, 'So you're the new vet then, are you?' Everyone in the town immediately knew who she was, it was like something out of James Herriot, but the down-side.

I suppose we'll probably stay where we are for the moment, but I can definitely see us moving within the next year or so. I think most new graduates tend to move jobs a few times before settling down somewhere long term.

Saturday 21 June

Bloody busy morning surgery again, which I ended up doing single-handedly, as usual. I always seem to be on with Keith on Saturdays, which tends to mean that I might as well be on my own. This is a rough summary of what we each did this morning:

	Joe	*Keith*
9.00 a.m.	two dog boosters	first cup of tea
	off-colour rabbit	
	itchy West Highland white	
9.30 a.m.	vomiting cat	second cup of tea,
	cat booster and worming	shuffles papers

guinea pig with mites
10.00 a.m. re-examine lame dog   puts on white coat
mad old lady with perfectly finally sees first
 healthy Yorkie   client, coughing
dog booster   dog
cat with bite wound
10.45 a.m. go out to two farm calls   has third cup of tea
and goes home

I wouldn't mind if it was my weekend on call but as he's on, he should do at least half the work if not most of it. Whenever it's the other way round and I'm on call and he's just in on Saturday morning, he does even less, saying that the second person only need do anything if the first vet is too busy.

I suppose I should count myself lucky though, because Keith is an angel to work with compared to some vets I've met in the past. There was one particular one I remember from one of the practices where I was a trainee before I qualified. His name was Derek and he was one of the worst vets I've ever known. He was a big, overweight York-shireman, who always dressed in horrible, tight check shirts, and cords that barely made it around his enormous girth.

Not only was he really lazy, but also he showed a complete lack of care for the animals he treated, partly because he was scared of them, I think. I saw him on quite a few occasions trying to deal with nervous or slightly aggressive animals by hitting them on the nose with a pen or a ruler. This just made the animals worse and he would turn round to the owners and say that he couldn't treat their animal because it was too dangerous. Luckily there were other vets around to show me how to deal properly with nervous and aggressive animals so I didn't end up following Derek's example.

Lots of clients refused to see him, because he was not only a bad vet and very bad with animals, but he could also be incredibly rude to clients. I saw him once sit in the office at one minute past seven, when evening surgery had officially finished, and refuse to see a client who had rushed in with a really sick dog as soon as she could. He said, in a voice easily loud enough to be heard in the waiting room, 'The bloody silly woman should have got here on time. If she wants to be seen, she can pay the out-of-hours emergency fee, but otherwise it'll have to wait until tomorrow because I'm off home.'

I don't know how vets like him get away with what they do. If I was a client and the vet spoke to me like that, or hit my dog because it growled at him, I'd certainly never go back again. What was strange was, that although most of the clients hated him and refused to see him, he had a small band of loyal clients who wouldn't ever see anybody else. I suppose for every different vet, however rude or incompetent, there will always be some clients who think they are the best thing ever.

Tuesday 24 June

Eric is looking really bad. He went downhill over the weekend, and we may have to think about putting him to sleep soon if he doesn't start to pick up. It's not fair to leave him in the state he's in. He's just standing in the stable, head down, with liquid diarrhoea pouring out of him. He's getting more dehydrated and weaker by the day. Miss Roberts is really upset because I think she knows what is coming. I had quite a long chat with her yesterday and she told me that she'd had the horse since she was twelve and he's been such a great friend for so long. She's not a typical horsy owner, she always turns up in jeans and a trendy jacket, not jodhpurs and riding boots. I don't think she's ridden him for years, the teenage girlie horse craze has passed, but she still obviously loves him and looks after him really well.

I'm not looking forward to having to tell her that it'd be best to put him to sleep, and even less actually to have to do it. I've never put a horse down, so not only will it be traumatic because of how upset the owner will be, but I'll also be nervous because I don't want to make a mess of the final minutes of her beloved horse's life.

Wednesday 25 June

Toby rang up last night. He's organizing a group holiday to France for the middle of July, which sounds great. I spoke to Emma about it and as long as we can both get the time off, I think we're going to go. It'll be wonderful to have a couple of weeks away and see everyone from university again. We're going camping on the west coast, down near Biarritz, which is a great area. I spent most of my summers while I was at university travelling around and surfing down there so I know it pretty well. I can't wait!

Thursday 26 June

1.15 p.m. I had to put Eric down this morning. It went OK, thankfully, but it was still a really upsetting and stressful experience.

Miss Roberts rang up after morning surgery and said that she'd discussed it with her father, who helps to look after the horse, and they'd both decided it would be best if they didn't let him suffer on any more.

As I'd never put a horse to sleep before I asked Ian for a bit of guidance, as there are quite a few different methods for doing it.

'I usually give them a bottle of Somulose in the vein,' he said, while he was preparing to go out TB testing. 'Some people shoot them but a lot of owners really don't like that, even though it's the quickest and kindest way to do it.'

If it works, I thought. I've seen a couple of animals shot

incorrectly and it wasn't a mistake that I'd like to make. It's really unpleasant and the animal suffers, as the gun has to be reloaded and fired again. However, one cow I saw shot hardly noticed as the bullet passed through her skull, narrowly missing the vital spot. She merely raised her head as if to say 'what was that noise?' and then carried on grazing, oblivious to the small hole smoking in her forehead. Horses are much more nervous, though, and unlikely to stand still if you have to have a second attempt, so I was relieved to hear Ian's advice. An injection sounded much easier and less dangerous than a gun.

When I arrived Miss Roberts was in tears and said her farewell to the horse in the stable. She didn't want to see her old friend killed, which was understandable. Her father, a quiet man of about fifty, dressed in a sober jumper and cords, led the horse down to the chosen spot where a hole had been dug for its grave. I drew up the required dose of the lethal injection and prepared the site on the horse's neck. Horses' veins are big and very easy to find, so I was able to slip the needle in without any difficulty (no repeat of that horrible dog euthanasia a month ago, thankfully). I drew back to check that I was in the vein, and after seeing the blood enter the syringe, I slowly pushed the plunger in.

I was unsure as to what to expect the horse to do. I'd heard stories of horses becoming excited and lashing out, but all that happened was that it dropped like a stone to the grass. It happened so fast that I hadn't injected all the drug, so I had to kneel down and finish the injection on the ground. Mr Roberts had been holding his head, and as he collapsed to the ground he bent down and said goodbye with a tear in his eye. It was all over within a few seconds – much to my relief. Although I failed to cure him of the salmonella, at least I managed to end his suffering in a painless and dignified manner.

I often think that putting animals to sleep is one of the most important services that vets provide, and helps to cure more pain and suffering than an awful lot of medicine and surgery. It makes me think about humans who are suffering with terminal illnesses, and the pain they have to endure in their last days or even months. With an animal in that situation we can just say, 'Right, there's no chance of the animal recovering, and they're suffering, so the best thing would be to put them out of their misery,' but with humans that's not done. Although the doctor may know that the patient is going to die a painful and lingering death, they can't release them and let them go in a quick and dignified way. They have to suffer on to the bitter end.

I understand the problems with legalizing euthanasia in humans and the worry that it will be exploited and misused, but I still believe there is a case, in selected instances, where it would be the right thing to do.

Sunday 29 June

7.15 p.m. Lovely relaxing weekend off. On Friday afternoon I took the grassboard out and had a really good session on it. I managed to do some excellent jumps and went down some difficult terrain. The only real problem at the moment is the weight, which is a bit restrictive when you're trying to do big jumps and things, so I went back to Peter Bullock and asked if he could make me a set of axles from aluminium instead of steel. He said that it shouldn't be a problem, if he can get hold of some suitable metal.

Today, the surf was reasonable, so Emma and I went in for a while. Tim came up from Bristol, which was good. I've known Tim for about five years, originally through the surf club at Bristol University, and we've been on quite a few surfing holidays together over the years. I asked him if he wanted to come to France with us next month but he said that he'd already agreed to go off somewhere with his girl-friend Nicky, so he couldn't come. He was pretty pissed off, but said his life wouldn't be worth living if he cancelled his holiday with Nicky. That's what happens when you get serious with a girlfriend, it'll be wedding bells and sprogs before long I should think. You wouldn't catch me missing out on a surf trip for a woman!

7.40 p.m. Ouch! Emma's just read my last entry and she's got my arm behind my back. Ow! She's just said that if I don't apologize for the last entry in writing, she'll break my arm and do something nasty to a vulnerable part of my lower body. OK, OK, I'll do it!

I am very sorry about what I wrote earlier, and I would not hesitate to sacrifice any surf trip to be with my beloved Emma.

Phew, thank God for that, I've got my arm back.

8.03 p.m. She's gone out to walk the dogs. I hearby withdraw my last statement, and reiterate the fact that surfing comes before . . . Oh, no! She's back! Now be reasonable, Em. No! Not that!
Aaaaahhhh!!!

July

Tuesday 1 July

Ricky, the dog with the bottom full of stones, came in again today. Mr Norman said that he'd been fine for a couple of weeks, but now the swelling was back and he was in a lot of pain again. I looked at his back end and the swelling was even bigger than it had been before. When I touched it, Ricky yelped and had a little nip at me.

'That's not like Ricky at all,' said Mr Norman, patting Ricky's muzzle. 'He must be hurting real bad for him to do that. Isn't there anything you can do to solve the problem once and for all, because I can't keep bringing him back every couple of weeks, it's just not fair on the poor old boy, is it?'

'Well, I've been giving it some thought since you last came in,' I replied, 'and there is an operation to repair the hernia that we could try. It's not without a few risks, but I really don't think we've got much choice. We can't leave him like this and, as you said, it's not fair on him to keep bringing him in to have it cleaned out every few weeks.'

We discussed the operation, which involved placing some deep sutures between the muscles of his back end and tightening them up to close the defect in the muscles where the hernia was pushing through. I explained the main risks were post-operative infection, and the possibility that I might damage the nerves supplying the anal sphincter during the operation, which could leave him unable to control his motions. In the end we decided it was worth the possible risks, and we booked him in for the operation next week.

I rang the BBC, and they're going to come and film the op. It'll be great if it works, because it should completely cure Ricky's problem. It'll also be good to get some decent surgery on camera as well. I just hope I don't make a mess of the operation because it's probably the trickiest thing I've tried so far.

Wednesday 2 July

6.15 p.m. I had an interesting case this afternoon. A woman brought in a pair of tortoises which had not been right since coming out of hibernation this spring. The owner was a really likeable lady called Mrs Powell. I think she comes from Spain or Portugal, but she married someone from this area and has lived here for years. She was very smartly dressed in a dark blouse and skirt, with heavy gold jewellery.

'They are not eating correctly,' she said, in a very mixed continental/Devon accent. 'Bluebell, this one, is really not herself. Normally she runs around the garden at this time of year, but she is really quiet and slow.'

I picked up Bluebell, the larger of the pair, and gave her a general check over. I've seen a few tortoises since I qualified, but not many, so I was feeling a little unsure of exactly what to look for and what I could do if I found a problem.

Bluebell and her male friend, Billy, both looked in reasonable condition, but it was hard to tell much, because of all the enclosing shell. I vaguely remembered some lectures that we had had on tortoises, and some of the information was drifting back. One of the techniques that had been demonstrated was listening to their chests using a stethoscope and towel.

'I'm just going to have a quick listen,' I said to Mrs Powell, who watched as I placed a towel over the shell and pressed the end of the stethoscope on to it. I was half expecting to hear a typical dog- or cat-type regular, loud heart, but I really couldn't make out any distinct noises. I was sure this was how the lecturer had demonstrated it, and he'd said we should be able to clearly hear the heart and breathing sounds.

'Her chest sounds fine,' I told Mrs Powell, telling myself that the absence of any wheezes or gurgles must mean there was nothing too serious going on inside, even if I wasn't entirely convinced that my auscultation technique was 100 per cent correct.

At this point I decided that rather than continue to rely on sketchy, half-remembered lecture notes, it would be best to consult a textbook for a few more ideas as to what I could do next. I excused myself, saying that I had just got to check a cat out the back, and went to find the ever-useful *Manual of Exotic Pets*.

After a quick flick through the relevant chapter, the old lecture memories started to come back. I remembered that one good method of determining a tortoise's general state of health was to compare its weight to the length of its shell. There was a chart in the book showing the ideal weight against length of shell, so all I had to do was weigh the tortoises and measure them and I would have a good idea if they were underweight or not.

I returned to the consulting room and tried to act as if this was what I had been planning to do all along.

'I'm just going to compare their weights to their lengths. That will give us a pretty good indication of their general state of health, and tell us if we need to do anything or not,' I told Mrs Powell as confidently as I could. I hadn't quite worked out exactly what I was going to do if they were underweight, but one step at a time I thought.

The resulting measurements and weights showed that both of the tortoises were in fact quite severely underweight. I excused myself again and had another look through the textbook, before returning to Mrs Powell.

'It's a tricky situation really,' I explained. 'They're both underweight, which is why they're off colour, but it's not going to be that simple to get them eating again. The only thing I can really try to help them put on a bit of weight is an injection of vitamins, which may just kick start them and get them going.'

I gave both tortoises a small injection of multi-vitamins

and asked Mrs Powell to pop them back in a week or so to see how they are getting on.

I enjoy dealing with exotic and unusual animals like tortoises, but I do wish we'd been taught a bit more about them at vet school. I feel a bit out of my depth sometimes, and I'm not always sure I'm doing the animals any good with my treatment. Experience is the only way to get better, though, so with luck I will start to improve my knowledge and be able to offer some useful treatment for animals like these. Relying on a sneaky look at a textbook is all very well, but it can't inspire too much confidence in the owner when the vet is nipping in and out to look things up all the time. I suppose it's better to admit that you aren't 100 per cent sure about something, swallow your pride and look it up, than to bluff your way through and get it wrong.

Saturday 5 July

8.15 p.m. On call all weekend. I've just been to see an ill cat at the surgery. The phone rang as I was out on the grassboard, and I had a lengthy discussion about whether or not I needed to see the cat, via my mobile phone, while lying in a mud-filled hollow clutching at my knee. When the phone rang, I was startled and veered horribly off course, colliding painfully with a large stone. It was all I could do to stifle a loud moan as I talked to the owner.

In the end I decided that the cat probably did need seeing, so I arranged to meet the owner, a Mrs Bloom, at the surgery in ten minutes. That just about gave me time to change out of my very muddy grassboarding gear (which consists of an old and ripped pair of tracksuit bottoms, my snowboarding boots and an old check shirt) and clean the worst of the mud off my face before she turned up.

Mrs Bloom was a well-dressed, middle-aged woman and she pulled up into the car park in an expensive-looking Japanese sports car (no concessions on the call-out fee for her, I thought). The cat, an ancient Siamese called Tululah, had been off colour all day and hadn't eaten or drunk since last night. She looked dehydrated and generally ill, although her temperature was normal. Signs of ongoing kidney failure were very evident. She was thin, due to muscle wasting, and her breath smelt of chronic renal failure. I guessed that her sudden deterioration was probably associated with this problem, so I treated her accordingly (fluids, antibiotics and an anabolic steroid injection). I hope that will be sufficient to get her back to normal again, but I told Mrs Bloom that the long-term outlook was pretty poor and that the only thing that could save her would be a kidney transplant, and they just aren't done on animals.

9.30 p.m. Calving at Brown's, damn!

10.20 p.m. Not too bad. One live calf coming backwards which just needed re-arranging and pulling hard. I actually didn't mind going out because it's such a nice evening. I love these summer evenings, when it's light until 10 p.m. It was really beautiful out in the field where this cow was, overlooking the sea, with the sun setting on the horizon. I may get frustrated with living out in the sticks occasionally, but evenings like tonight make up for an awful lot of missed nights out in lively pubs and cinemas.

Sunday 6 July

9.30 a.m. I was woken up by some stupid bloke at 6.00 this morning. I answered the phone, expecting a calving or something else pretty urgent, but no, this bloke was just worried because his cat was coughing. I asked him how long the cat had been doing this and he said, 'Oh, for a few days now.' Why does he have to wait until the middle of the night before deciding he needs to ring the vet? What's wrong with bringing the cat down to the surgery, or at least ringing at a reasonable hour? It wasn't as if the cat was very ill either, and when I told him that I could see it, but it would cost him about £50, he said, 'Oh, well, I think I'll leave it for now and see how she is in the morning.'

People just assume that because there is a twenty-four-hour emergency service, there is a vet sitting happily by the phone day and night waiting to give out advice and cheerfully discuss minor ailments in the small hours. What people don't realize is that there is one vet on all weekend and, like most other normal people, we quite appreciate the little things in life such as sleep! People like that really wind me up!

8.30 p.m. Emma's come over and we're having a nice romantic meal together in a minute, so I'm bound to get called out halfway through.

8.45 p.m. I can't believe it! I've got to go out to a horse with suspected colic! That is just so typical of the kind of weekend I'm having. I spent the whole day going back and forth to the surgery seeing off-colour dogs and vomiting cats, so I was looking forward to having a nice quiet night at home. No such luck!

9.50 p.m. Horse fixed, dinner burnt, Emma annoyed, Joe in very bad mood!

Monday 7 July

8.45 a.m. The BBC have arrived to film Ricky's operation this morning. Sarah, the usual director, has been replaced by Amanda, as Sarah is off filming something else at the moment (*Holiday Reps*, I think). Both Emma and I have really got to like Sarah, so I hope she returns after her jaunt to the Canaries or wherever it is she's gone to. I'm sure Amanda will be just as nice, but we were getting used to talking to Sarah on film and it may take a little while to get that same relationship going with a new director. When we first started being filmed we were both quite nervous and didn't relax or talk fluidly in front of the cameras, but as we've got more used to it, and got to know Sarah, it's become much easier to be natural.

1.30 p.m. A stressful, but pretty satisfying morning. The operation went really well, much better than I expected.

I did it with a surgery textbook open on the table next to me so that I could refer to it as I went along. It was useful in helping me identify exactly which muscles and nerves were which, something vital to the success of the operation. It involved stitching three muscles together to repair the defect in the muscle wall, which usually supports each side of the anus. In these cases, this muscle wall has deteriorated and allowed a pouch of rectum to push through under the skin. The main difficulties are avoiding all the big important nerves which run through the area and the fact that all the stitching is done about two inches in, making it very tricky to tie the knots well.

It took about an hour in all and, although everything went well, the real proof that it worked won't come until he's gone for at least a few months without a recurrence of the hernia, and even then it could still break down later on. Still, I'm pleased with the result, and it should look good on film. It was a bit of a risk telling the BBC about the op because, if it hadn't gone to plan and I'd made a mess of it, not only would Ricky have suffered but the whole nation would have seen my incompetence!

I think Trude, the Norwegian vet who is also being filmed for this series, suffered a lot from the BBC showing her making a hash of an injection in *Vet's School*. Although it was a simple mistake that all vets have made at some time or other (I know I've done it on several occasions), the public leapt on it as a sign of general incompetence rather than seeing it as part of the learning experience we all go through. I mean, she was only a student at the time, and the whole point of training is to make mistakes and learn from them. I bet she's never done that again, unlike most vets.

I've done a couple of injections, usually boosters, when I've either injected straight through the skin as she did, or the needle has come off the syringe and the contents have leaked out that way. It's always a bit of a dilemma if the owners don't notice – you can either ignore it (but then have to worry all day that the animal didn't get the right dose and might get ill as a result), or own up and accept the humiliation and lost respect. I usually end up admitting to it because it's just not worth the risk, and owners are usually pretty understanding.

Tuesday 8 July

1.00 p.m. Ricky went home this morning looking well. Even if it doesn't work in the long term, it's given him some temporary relief at any rate. It must be such a nice feeling for him to wake up from the anaesthetic with such a large painful mass gone. Dogs are so trusting. It amazes me what they let us do to them without really putting up any resistance. They just assume that what we're doing is best for them and let us get on with it. There are the exceptions, of course, but in general most dogs see us humans as the equivalent of their pack leader and therefore do what we ask of them without question.

8.15 p.m. Emma over, going to pub.

12.30 a.m. Ow! We were playing our silly 'let's hide from the dogs' game just now when we took them out for a drunken walk to the sea, and I tried to hide Emma in a ditch. She got very unreasonable and punched me – I mean, how was I to know the ditch was waist deep in muddy water? She says that the stain will never wash out of her favourite top. I think I may be sleeping with the mutts tonight.

Wednesday 9 July

8.40 a.m. Hungover!

11.30 a.m. The BBC want to film me grassboarding as I've got some time off this afternoon. The aluminium prototype isn't ready yet so I'll have to use the old steel one, which is a shame because I want it to look as impressive as possible. Perhaps someone from a large snowboarding company will see it on TV and then offer me hundreds of thousands of pounds for the idea. Well, maybe fifty quid anyway!

I hope the hangover has improved by the time I have to strap myself in and launch myself down some hills this afternoon, because at the moment my head feels like there's a small, angry Staffordshire bull terrier inside!

6.30 p.m. The grassboarding was excellent. I took the new ramp up to the park in Bideford and did some jumps, which will look pretty good on film, I hope. The camera crew were finding it all a bit hard to take seriously. There they were, engaged to come and film a serious documentary about a vet, and they end up lying on some damp grass next to a home-made ramp, filming the vet throwing himself over it on an overgrown skateboard! Sometimes I do think I have gone slightly mad, but I suppose anyone who's invented a new sport must have been through the same kind of thing. I bet the person who invented football must have stopped one day and said to himself, 'What the bloody hell am I doing, kicking an inflated cow's bladder around this empty field?'

Friday 11 July

I had one of the most upsetting cases of my career so far this morning. Luckily the BBC went yesterday, because they would have made a difficult case even worse if they'd been here. It was bad enough without them around.

It was a dog that the owners wanted putting to sleep

because it had started weeing in the house. They didn't want to bring him into the practice, so I drove out to their house after morning surgery had finished. It was a nice old detached building on the main road of a small village, with a large garden sloping down to the river. The owner was a woman of about forty, called Mrs Turner. She greeted me holding a dripping mop and carrying a bucket.

'He's done it again, the poor old boy,' she said, as she ushered me into the kitchen. 'He just can't seem to control himself anymore.'

At that point a healthy looking, elderly chocolate Labrador wandered into the room and greeted us both with a wag of the tail and friendly lick. I assumed initially that this couldn't be Sam, the dog in question, because he looked so well, but when he wandered back towards the open door, Mrs Turner called him and I realized that this was in fact the dog that they wanted put to sleep.

'He looks pretty well in general, for an older dog,' I said, as I knelt next to him and looked him over. 'Is there anything else wrong with him, or is it just the weeing in the house?'

'It's just the weeing, I'm afraid. It's ruined the carpets in the lounge, and the whole house stinks.' She looked fondly at the dog, but I could see that when it came down to it, the carpets came first.

'He is nearly twelve, and he's had a good life,' she said, obviously feeling as if she should justify her decision to me, 'and we don't think that he's at all happy. It's the best thing for him.'

Best thing for you, I thought.

'Couldn't you keep him out in a kennel?' I suggested.

'Oh no, he's too old to be out in the cold. He wouldn't understand why we'd put him out there. We've made up our minds and I think we're doing the best for him.'

I suppose she had a point, but I still felt as though they were taking the easy option and had convinced themselves they were doing the right thing. It wasn't my place to argue though, it was really their decision, and if I didn't do it then they would only go somewhere else.

I fetched the injection from the car and asked Mrs Turner to sit down with Sam and hold him still. He sat perfectly as I clipped the hair up his front leg, looking at his owner enquiringly, but not in any way concerned. The trust in his face was absolute. He completely trusted his owner, and the thought didn't even cross his mind that we might be planning to do anything to harm him.

I nearly stopped and took him home with me, but I knew it wouldn't be the right thing to do. It wouldn't have been fair on Sam or the owner.

I picked up the syringe and pushed the needle through the brown skin and into the vein below. He flinched and looked up for reassurance from Mrs Turner, but there was still no doubt or fear in his mind – his owner was there to look after him, why would she hurt him?

I injected the lethal blue solution. As the cold drug entered his blood stream, I could see a moment of terrible realization on his face. He looked accusingly at me and then in disbelief at Mrs Turner, before sinking into unconsciousness.

I turned away to hide the tears in my eyes. I've never felt so upset putting an animal to sleep before. It was the betrayal of all that trust and dedication.

It was also because I really felt that he didn't need to be put down. The owners just found that he had become inconvenient and had decided to get rid of him. That dog would have done anything for them, and they wouldn't even put up with a bit of urine in the lounge.

I looked at Mrs Turner and saw her look sorrowfully at Sam's unmoving body. I think she was genuinely upset, but still thought she'd done the right thing. I suppose some people just have different priorities. I'm all in favour of not letting an animal suffer unnecessarily if it's ill or just ancient, but I don't agree with people taking advantage of the fact that they can have their animals put to sleep and using any sign of old age or infirmity as an excuse to get rid of an inconvenient animal.

I took Sam's body back to the surgery and placed him in the freezer. A van comes and collects all the frozen bodies once a week and takes them to the pet crematorium, where they are cremated together. Some people like to pay a premium and have their pet individually cremated so they can have their ashes back in a small urn. Somehow I didn't think Mrs Turner would want to spend the extra on something like that, she'd be more likely to spend the money on new carpets.

Saturday 12 July

1.40 p.m. I went out to see Mrs Powell, the tortoise lady, this morning. She said that she had some wonderful news, and it would be best explained if I came to the house. I finished morning surgery (with Ian, so I actually got away at a decent time) and drove up to her place in Bideford.

The house is a large bungalow set back in a well-tended garden. As I walked up the path to the front door, a large pet rabbit hopped past and disappeared into a greenhouse at the end of the garden, and two wild squirrels ran off from the front steps of the house where they'd been feeding from a bowl of nuts. I knocked on the front door and Mrs Powell ushered me through into the living room.

Sitting on the expensive-looking carpet were Bluebell and Billy, both contentedly nibbling on a small pile of cherries and lettuce leaves.

'How are they both?' I asked Mrs Powell

'Oh, very well, they're both eating well and look much happier. In fact we had a bit of a surprise yesterday – Bluebell laid some eggs!'

She took me over to the sideboard, where there was a

small plastic box filled with sand sitting next to a slightly larger metal box which had several knobs and lights on top.

'This is our incubator,' she said proudly. 'My husband is an electrical engineer, so once we suspected that she might be having some more eggs, he built this.'

'Has she had eggs before, then?' I asked.

'Yes, last year we had some but the incubator which we borrowed from someone broke down and the eggs never hatched. It's very difficult to get live young, the temperature has to be just right, and very constant.'

She opened the lid of the new incubator and scraped off a little sand to reveal the tops of three small white eggs.

'My husband designed this to keep the eggs at exactly the correct temperature, and it's got a sensor so that when the eggs start to hatch an alarm will go off.'

'No! You're having me on,' I replied, thinking that a home-made incubator was one thing, but surely a built-in egg-hatching alarm was stretching the bounds of feasibility just a little.

'No, no really, it works, look.' She flicked a switch marked 'hatch sensor on' and then waggled a finger in the sand. For a second nothing happened, and then the silence was broken by the sound of a digital alarm clock coming from the metal box.

'I'm impressed!' I really appreciate this kind of thing, it strikes a chord with the inventor in me. 'When are they due to hatch?' I asked, carefully touching one of the exposed eggs.

'Oh, not until the end of August, I think. It will be very exciting if they are alive.'

'You must let me know when it happens, I'd love to see them when they've hatched.'

I left in high spirits. I really like Mrs Powell, and the tortoises are great. I've not really had much contact with them in the past, so it's a real learning experience for me. I was surprised to see how fast they can move. When I left, they were chasing each other around the room at a very impressive rate!

Maybe I'll become a specialist tortoise vet!

Monday 14 July

We're going on holiday in four days' time. Hooray! It's going to be fantastic! No more squeezing anal glands and talking to miserable owners for two whole weeks.

I'm really getting fed up with some bits of my job, especially morning surgery. I'm not at my best first thing anyway, and the prospect of starting each day with an hour and a half of open surgery does nothing to improve my mood! If we had some form of rota where we took it in turns to do morning surgery, or go out on visits, or start operating, it would be much better. I can't see that happening though, Keith's too keen on his morning tea, and Ian's a large-animal vet at heart and tries to avoid small-animal consulting where possible. I know that I shouldn't be whingeing because they are my bosses after all, and they can choose what they want to do, but I am getting a bit annoyed by the whole set-up.

Tuesday 15 July

A much better day today. Rectum Ricky (as the BBC crew have called him) came in to have the stitches taken out of the skin today. The wound has healed up fine and there's no sign of any infection or recurrence of the hernia. The internal stitches, which are holding everything together inside, will gradually dissolve over the next few months, by which time the muscles should have knitted together to form a permanent repair.

Mr Norman is very pleased with the outcome, he said that Ricky is like a new dog. I just hope that it doesn't all break down in the next few weeks, but the fact that it's lasted this long without a problem is a good sign.

*

The farm work has really dropped off over the last few months, mainly because the dairy cows are all out at pasture. An awful lot of their health problems, such as bad feet and mastitis, tend to come in the winter when they're housed in dirty cubicles. We do see some cows in the summer, but it's mainly the odd case of milk fever, or a calving, or a nasty summer mastitis. Most of the farmers don't bother with routine pregnancy checks and fertility work through the summer, because the calving and associated veterinary work happens in the winter months. As a result, we're pretty quiet on the farm side of things at present. It's counterbalanced to a large degree by the increase in small-animal work in the summer. We tend to see a lot of holiday-makers, which makes us busier, but in general small-animal practice tends to be busier in the summer. I'm not quite sure why this is, perhaps it's because more people are out walking their dogs (lameness, bites, etc.) and cats are out scrapping (abscesses, ripped claws, etc.). A lot of people buy animals in the summer, so we see them for their first vaccinations and neutering as well.

In general, most older, mixed practices are becoming more and more small-animal orientated as the large-animal work declines. Witten Lodge, for example, used to be a mainly large-animal practice with only a small percentage of its work being small-animal. Now we do only about 40 per cent large-animal, and according to Ian, it's getting less each year. The reasons are complex, but much of the drop in work must be due to the loss of all the small farms, which are being replaced by big, more self-sufficient farms, where the stockman does a lot of the work once done by the vet. Also, with problems such as BSE, and disappearing subsidies affecting farmers' profits, vets' bills are bound to be cut back on as much as possible.

Some practices have decided that large-animal work is no longer worth the effort and have pulled out completely. A lot of areas are being served by dedicated large-animal practices which offer high standards and work closely with the big farms. I think this is the logical progression for vets, and in a few years mixed practice may well be a thing of the past. It will be a shame, though, because one of the great attractions of being a vet is the variety of the work, and that's going to be lost if all vets end up as specialists.

Thursday 17 July

6.30 p.m. Finished for two weeks! I've just emptied all the vet stuff out of the back of my car. The wonderful Joe's Vet Box is in a bit of a state after several months of absorbing horrible wet leaks from my boots and things. The wood has gone mouldy and smells pretty grim. I'm going to leave it in the garden while I'm away to bake in the sun and dry out (knowing the English weather it'll probably rain the whole time and it'll end up in an even worse state, if that's possible).

Blackie, the devil cat, is being fed by the couple next door. They should get on well!

8.15 p.m. Dulverton All packed and ready to go. The poor little practice car is loaded up to the hilt with surfboards, a tent, sleeping bags and food.

The dogs are staying with one of Emma's farm clients. Her parents refused to have them again on the grounds that they like their garden the way it is and have no desire to have any more large holes dug in it, which is fair enough, I suppose.

Friday 18 July

10.15 a.m. Another emotional farewell with the mutts. We had to leave them in a stable on the farm, and as we drove away we could see them poking their heads out over the door, whining pitifully. It was really upsetting because we wanted to tell them that it was OK and that we'd come back for them in two weeks. For all they knew, we could have been abandoning them, never to return.

We've only been gone half an hour and already I miss their stupid licking muzzles!

4.15 p.m. Portsmouth Met Toby and everyone. Boarding the ferry in about an hour. I can't wait to get there and see the sea, I hope we get good surf!

6.25 p.m. *Pride of Cherbourg* We're off! Two weeks of surfing, drinking and sunbathing, and no morning surgeries!

August

Sunday 3 August

9.30 p.m. Dulverton What a journey! We left Biarritz yesterday morning and aimed to get on the evening ferry last night, but unfortunately the weather was too bad so the crossing was cancelled. We had to wait all night in the car park, trying to get some sleep in the car, which considering the size of the car was pretty optimistic! In the end we got a ferry first thing this morning and finally got back here this afternoon. It's been a fantastic holiday though. The surf was brilliant, and the weather was pretty good for most of the time (except one night when we camped on the dunes and a massive storm came in from the sea and completely wiped out the tents!).

When we got back the first thing we did was to go and get the mutts. They were so pleased to see us – they wouldn't stop jumping up and licking our faces for about five minutes. Mrs Stewart, the farmer who looked after them, said they had been well behaved and had had an excellent time chasing rabbits with her pack of spaniels. She did say that Badger had howled for the first five nights though! Poor old Badge, he's so sensitive and worries all the time. Pan just chills out and doesn't mind what's going on, whereas Badger gets really upset if he gets told off or something strange happens.

All the time we've been away I've been thinking things over and I've come to a big decision – I'm going to hand in my notice and look for a new job!

Although I've really enjoyed working in Bideford, and I like the people, I think it's time for a change and some new challenges. One of the best things about being a vet is that there are always lots of jobs available and unemployment isn't really a risk. So I can afford to make the decision to leave this job and look for a new one without worrying too much about not being able to find a new job.

I feel I need to move to a new practice to start learning

some more skills and develop as a vet, rather than stay here and just carry on as I am. I've learnt a lot in the last year but, because it's quite a small, country practice, I haven't got to do or see much really high-powered operating, which is what I'm mostly interested in. I feel I've got good, basic all-round knowledge, but to progress I need to move to somewhere new.

It's going to be awful telling Ian, because I think they would like me to stay on for another year. Not because I'm anything special, but just for the stability, so all the clients, especially the farmers, aren't constantly seeing new and different vets all the time. I really like Ian, and Keith's not too bad on his good days, so it's going to be quite upsetting. I hope they don't just turn around and say, 'Oh, you off then, are you? Bye then, nice meeting you.'

Emma's also thinking of leaving her practice, for pretty much the same reasons as me. She's really into surgery and might even consider applying for a residency back at the vet school in Langford, near Bristol. One of the vets there, who Emma got on with really well, rang her up a few weeks back and told her there was a vacancy for a small-animal soft-tissue surgeon coming up, and that he thought she would stand a good chance of getting it.

I think it would be great if she went for it. Although it would mean a few years of pretty crap pay, she would get so much good experience and job satisfaction. The only worry is that soft-tissue residents tend to sleep with most of the final-year students, but I think I can trust her!

I've got to pluck up the courage to break the news to Ian and Keith tomorrow. Not looking forward to it at all.

Monday 4 August

11.45 a.m. I've finished morning surgery, Ian's around. Now's the time to do it.

11.47 a.m. Bottled it! I was about to ask to speak to him when the phone rang, and I used that as an excuse to delay. It's not going to be that bad. No need to worry. Just tell him that you're leaving, what could be easier?

11.50 a.m. Hands shaking too much. Need a cup of tea to settle my nerves.

12.35 p.m. Well, the deed is done, I'm leaving at the end of the month. It didn't go exactly to plan though. In fact it was an absolute disaster. Just as I was about to ask if I could speak to Ian, he came up to me and said, 'Joe, can I just see you for a minute?'

He walked off to the main consulting room, as the office was busy with nurses, and I followed wondering what on earth he wanted to see me about. Maybe he was going to save me the effort of handing in my notice and sack me. But why? Perhaps he'd seen me on the grassboard and thought I was giving the practice a bad name.

As he started to talk, I could see that he was a bit nervous and on edge. I don't think that a pressurized situation such as sacking, or whatever was coming, is really Ian's forte, he's more of a non-confrontational type.

'Er, you've been with us for a year now,' he started, 'and we like to review salaries every twelve months. Therefore, we've decided to increase your salary this year to £16,500. I hope that's all right with you?'

Oh no! I thought. Here I am just about to hand in my resignation, and he's given me a pay rise. What a terrible bit of bad timing! There was no escaping what I had to do, though. I'd made my mind up and I had to go through with it.

'Er, yes, that's brilliant,' I replied slowly, conscious of the fact that I wasn't displaying the expected enthusiasm and gratitude that usually follow a generous pay rise. 'I'm really sorry, but I've decided that it's time for me to move on.'

I saw the surprise and disappointment register on Ian's usually passive face.

'Oh,' he said, sadly, and continued after a pause, 'We were hoping that you were planning to stay on for another year or two.'

'I'm really sorry, messing you around and everything. It's just that Emma's thinking of moving back to Bristol, and we want to get a house together and things.' I felt so guilty, like I was really letting him down. I could see he hadn't been expecting the news, and that it had come as a bit of a blow.

'When were you thinking of leaving, then?' he asked.

'Well, at the end of the month if that's OK.'

'Right, we'll have to get an advert in the *Vet Record* straight away,' he said.

And that was that. I had officially given in my notice, and in four weeks' time I'll be jobless, homeless and carless!

9.50 p.m. Emma's here, and we've just had a long talk about our future and what we want to do. She's decided to hand in her notice as well, and go for the job back at Langford.

I still feel really sad and guilty about leaving, it's almost like ending a relationship. I keep having doubts, thinking that maybe I'm being too hasty, and that I'll get my enthusiasm for the job back if I stick at it for a bit longer. I know deep down that I've done the right thing though. I need to move on and try something new and different, otherwise I'll end up stagnating away here and never leave.

10.30 p.m. Blackie, the devil cat, has just dragged a semi-alive mouse in. Poor thing, little does it know that it's destined for eternity in the clutches of the feline anti-Christ. That cat is one thing that I will definitely not miss when I leave!

Tuesday 5 August

Everyone at work knows I'm leaving. Keith hasn't really said anything, but I assume Ian has told him. I ended up telling

Jamie, and once one of the nurses knows something, then the others are as good as told. Even Sue the receptionist knew within a minute of arriving this afternoon. I'm going to miss the nurses and Sue, they've been really good while I've been here, and helped me through my first year as a vet. Having decent, friendly nurses makes such a difference. It would be very hard to get through the first months as a newly qualified vet without their tactful support. The first few operations I did would have been even more of a shambles than they were if it weren't for Helen and Taryn giving me tips and pointing me roughly in the right direction – 'Yes, that pink bit there. No! Not that one. No! Don't cut that! OK, OK. Calm down. Just put the clamps on it and it'll stop bleeding in a minute. Wait, I think I'd better get Ian . . . '

Thursday 7 August

1.30 p.m. We actually had some farm work today. It's been dead for weeks, just the odd calving and stuff, but today both Ian and I were busy out on farms all morning. I didn't have the courage to tell any of the farmers about my impending departure. It's not that I think they'll be terribly upset at losing me as a vet, it's more the disruption of getting used to a new vet. I like to think that I've built up a pretty good relationship with most of them, and I will be sorry to leave most of them (there are certainly a few exceptions, such as Brian Hill's mud pit).

I had an awful visit just before lunch. I had to go and see a farrowing pig which was having difficulty producing any piglets. It is owned by a retired teacher called Mr Loveridge, who has a smallholding by the sea a few miles up the coast. I'd been there once before to see one of his calves. He's got about forty cows and their offspring, as well as two pedigree pigs and a couple of ponies.

I turned up and Mr Loveridge ushered me into the small pigsty, which was basically a corrugated iron tunnel filled with straw. Mr Loveridge is a large man of about fifty, with receding grey hair and the stern manner of an ex-teacher.

'I was rather hoping that Ian or Keith would come,' he said as we clambered into the pen where the large pink sow was laying, 'but I suppose we'll have to see what you can do.'

'I'll try my best,' I said, through gritted teeth.

'Yes, well, let's hope it's good enough. She's a very valuable pedigree you know. Do you know what breed she is?'

'Landrace,' I said, on the verge of telling him what he could do with his precious porcine pedigree.

Ignoring my answer (presumably because it was correct, and therefore gave him no opportunity to further belittle my knowledge) he moved towards the recumbent animal and gently tried to catch hold of her. As soon as he got up to her, she jumped to her feet with surprising agility and ran off to the far end of the pen. It took us a few minutes with the help of a large wooden board to get the pig cornered and fairly well restrained. Mr Loveridge held on to her while I examined her.

Inside, I could feel the cervix was almost closed. There was no way that any piglets were going to be delivered until it dilated.

I told Mr Loveridge, and suggested that the only course of action was to leave her and see what happened. There was nothing I could do to help dilate the cervix, and the only other option would be a caesar, an operation rarely, if ever, performed on pigs. The prospect of trying to anaesthetize and operate on a half-ton pig in a dirty pen was not a realistic one.

Mr Loveridge grumbled on, saying he wished he'd never called me out if all I was going to suggest was doing nothing, and that the cost of a visit was extortionate, and there must be something I could do. I thought that if it had been Ian or Keith who had come out and they had made the same suggestion, he would have accepted their advice, but as it was the young fresh-out-of-school vet, he wasn't going to listen to whatever I said, however correct.

4.20 p.m. I can't believe it! Mr Loveridge has just rung up and spoken to Ian to ask his advice because he wasn't happy with what I've told him. He said, 'I want you or Keith out here straight away. Next time I ask for a vet to see a pig, I want a vet who knows about pigs and not the tea boy!'

Tea boy! Just because I'm not fifty and grey he assumes I must be completely useless and know nothing. Ian and Keith are welcome to the arrogant, rude, narrow-minded pig-fancying pillock! I hope the pig charges him down and crushes him painfully to death in a pile of pedigree porcine slurry.

5.30 p.m. Ian went out and came to exactly the same conclusion as I did. He told Mr Loveridge that he would have to wait and see what happened or just cut his losses and shoot her, so that she didn't suffer any more. Even though it came from Ian, he still didn't really want to hear it, so he told Ian he was going to consult a friend who was a big pig farmer in Wiltshire and see what he said.

Ian was quite amused by the whole situation, and said there was nothing you could do for clients like him. If they aren't going to listen to your advice, then why do they bother to call you out in the first place?

Friday 8 August

10.00 a.m. Mr Loveridge has just rung up to demand a vet comes out and shoots the sow because there has been no progress overnight. He didn't mention his pig farmer friend, so I presume his advice was the same as ours. Ian's just gone out. I would have had trouble being civil to Mr Loveridge if I'd gone. Tea boy indeed!

12.35 p.m. Just read the *Veterinary Record* job section and I've seen something which might be suitable. It's for a chain of veterinary surgeries called Companion Care, a new company which is putting surgeries in pet superstores. I'm not sure what the job would be like, but the salary they quote is amazing: £30,000 plus car and housing allowance, which is nearly double what I'm on at the moment!

I might give them a ring and get some more details.

1.15 p.m. Interview next Thursday afternoon! I spoke to the personnel manager, and she gave me a brief outline of the job (fairly long hours, working solo in an in-store surgery, lots of good equipment and trained nurses). I asked whether the salary advertised would still be the same for someone like me, with only one year's experience, and she said that it probably would be. Thirty thousand pounds a year, imagine that!

She also said there were vacancies in Cardiff and Swansea, both of which wouldn't be too far from Emma if she gets the job at Langford. It sounds almost too good to be true (well, the pay does anyway).

7.30 p.m. On call tonight and all weekend. This'll teach me to go away on holiday!

Monday 11 August

Busy weekend. Lots of annoying holiday-makers with silly little dogs with very minor ailments, e.g. middle-aged caravanning couple with miniature Yorkshire terrier which has bruised pad!

I finally managed to get back to writing a bit more of my novel, which I have neglected over the last couple of months. I decided to get things moving so, after a few more odd finds in the surgery (empty human blood-transfusion bag, human endo-tracheal tube, etc.), Ben has his first encounter with one of Peter's victims, although he's still in the dark as to what's going on.

Ben slowly inched the calving rope over the unseen leg and pulled the loop tight above the fetlock. 'Right, that's got them, now it's just a matter of pulling it out,' he said cheerfully to Graham, the young stockman.

Ben had become a familiar face at Downend Farm, and got on well with Graham and his boss, Tony Hall. Graham was one of the new breed of stockmen, who had a diploma in agricultural science and applied his knowledge usefully to the everyday running of this large dairy farm.

Ben pieced together the calving jack and rested one end up against the cow's rump. Then he looped the free ends of the two calving ropes over the hooks on the jack and slowly worked the ratchet mechanism to take up the slack on the ropes.

'Take over here will you, Graham, I'm just going to make sure everything's coming OK inside,' he said, handing the jack over and washing his arm.

He felt inside and after some minor adjustments, the calf started to move through the birth canal as Graham increased the pressure from the jack. Soon the head and forelegs were showing and then, in one quick rush, the calf slid out and was lowered gently to the straw by Graham.

"Ee's a heifer,' announced Graham, obviously pleased with the outcome. He stood up and turned to face Ben, who was checking inside to ensure that the female calf had no brothers or sisters left behind. Just as Ben moved away, happy that the calf had been a single, the cow let loose a jet of watery brown faeces, which hit Graham squarely on the chest and covered his clean blue shirt.

Ben couldn't help but laugh as his friend picked himself up from the straw, stripping off the soaked shirt. 'That was superb,' he said, between fits of laughter. 'All over you. What a great aim that cow's got!'

'Yeah, wonderful!' agreed Graham, washing the worst of the mess from his face and arms. He turned to put his head under the cold tap and as he did so Ben stopped laughing.

'I didn't know that you'd had surgery Graham, what did you have done?' he asked.

'What are you talking about? I'm fine,' replied Graham, from underneath the cascade of cold water.

'But what's this wound on your back?' persisted Ben. 'There's a cut about four inches long with one, two, three, oh about eight stitches in it. Looks pretty fresh as well. I bet you got pissed as usual at the weekend and fell over on some glass or something, and now you're either too embarrassed to admit to it, or you were so drunk that you can't remember.'

Graham felt around and touched the wound, which was on the left-hand side of his back, just below his ribs.

'Bloody hell! What on earth?' He looked worriedly at Ben. 'I can't remember having this done. All I remember from Saturday night is getting really drunk after only a few pints and then waking up outside the pub, freezing cold, on Sunday morning. I thought I'd just fallen asleep there, I mean it wouldn't be the first time something like that has happened, would it? Look at what happened at the Young Farmers' Ball.'

Ben had been told many a story about Graham's legendary drinking and its amusing consequences. Apparently, at the ball, Graham had become so intoxicated that he'd fallen unconscious into a decorative fountain and had had to be rescued from hypothermia by some friends. Still, being too drunk to remember the evening was one thing, but ending

*up with a neat surgical scar on your back was a
different matter entirely – what on earth had he done
which could have needed such a major repair and
left him with no recollection of events?*

*'I think we'd better get you down to the hospital
and get this checked out,' said Ben as he cleaned up
his calving gear. He turned back to face Graham
but, as he did so, he saw the colour drain from the
stockman's face. Before Ben could reach out to
steady him, he collapsed on to the soft straw in an
unconscious heap.*

The excitement just keeps on coming! What'll happen next
is that Graham will be rushed to hospital suffering from
acute kidney failure, as of course the scar on his back is
from evil Peter stealing one of his kidneys. His other kidney
has been overloaded and a combination of that and some
post-operative infection has caused the collapse. I think he'll
just pull through, and together he and Ben will start to deduce
what has happened (with the help of love interest, Emily the
nurse).

Tuesday 12 August

Two bits of news from Emma. Firstly she has applied for the
job back at Langford, and secondly she's gone and got two
kittens!

She really scared me when I arrived at her place after
work today, because as I walked in she said, 'Joe, what do
you think about the patter of little feet?'

'Er, um, well, of course, er . . . ' I stammered nervously. I
do want babies eventually, but not right now. I didn't want
to be too negative, though, because if they were on the way,
I'd have to be enthusiastic for Emma's sake. 'So, er, little feet,
you say? Er, how? Er, when?'

'Just go upstairs and look in the spare room,' she replied

smiling. I relaxed a little – she was joking! Or was she? Perhaps there was a cot or a romper suit awaiting me in the spare room!

I opened the door and was greeted not by a pile of new baby equipment, but by two very cute little kittens.

'Thank God!' I said, as Emma followed me into the room. 'They're lovely. Where did they come from?'

'One of our farmers asked me if I would take them. I thought they would be good company for Charlie.' Charlie is Emma's three-legged cat who was found as a tiny kitten on a rubbish tip, with a mangled back leg. He'd obviously been abandoned and left there to die, but some kind passer-by had found him and taken him into the surgery in Kent where Emma worked for a few months after she qualified. The leg had to be amputated, and Emma took him on once he'd recovered from his ordeal.

We spent most of the evening playing with the new arrivals and trying to think up suitable names for them. In the end we decided to give them the worst cat names we could think of, so the little silver tabby one is Nigel and the ginger and white one is Brian!

Badger and Pan came upstairs to see them and were really good with them. Badger loves young animals of all kinds, and is very gentle and careful with them. He's the same with new-born calves and lambs, instead of eating them like Pan would, he licks them clean and generally mothers them.

Wednesday 13 August

10.40 p.m. Dulverton Interview tomorrow for Companion Care. I've got to drive all the way to a hotel in Portsmouth, have the interview, and then drive all the way back to do evening surgery in Bideford. I need a decent night's sleep.

1.30 a.m. Bugger! Can't sleep. Keep thinking about how vital it is for me to get a good night's sleep to do well at the interview. Try counting sheep.

2.15 a.m. Sheep no good, still wide awake.

2.32 a.m. Now Nigel and Brian have started meowing next door, little sods.

2.39 a.m. Fed the kittens, now surely I can get some sleep.

Thursday 14 August

7.00 a.m. What a terrible night. I think I got about two or three hours in, what with my pre-interview nerves and the bloody kittens! It's a good job I haven't got a three-hour drive followed by an important interview, another three-hour drive and then a busy evening surgery, isn't it!

11.30 a.m. Travelodge Hotel, Portsmouth I made it in one piece. Half an hour to wait before my interview. I can see a couple of other potential interviewees wandering around looking nervous. I need a cup of coffee.

1.05 p.m. McDonald's, Portsmouth I got offered the job! I can't believe it! Thirty thousand pounds plus housing and car allowances. The interview was with one of the partners of Companion Care, Peter Eville, who looked more like a high-powered businessman than a vet. He was only about thirty-two or three, and dressed smartly in a dark suit, with neatly styled hair and a briefcase. He met me in the hotel lobby and took me through to a small conference room. In the room was a large table covered in Companion Care leaflets and files. Against one wall was a large display board showing pictures of Companion Care surgeries inside and out. It all looked very impressive and well organized, a far cry from my interview at Witten Lodge, where I sat down with Ian and Keith in the half-decorated office and chatted informally over a cup of tea.

Peter Eville spent about half an hour telling me all about the way in which his company worked and how it was set up. Apparently he started off with his own practice soon after leaving college, then formed his own company providing vet services to abattoirs, and then in the last couple of years has started Companion Care, which is very much based on the way things are going in America.

Basically, what he and his partner are trying to do is set up a nationwide chain of high-quality practices in pet superstores. He assured me that they weren't trying to offer cheap, cut-price services, in fact they were really looking at the other end of the spectrum, the better-off clients who want to do everything possible for their animals and don't mind paying for it. They are trying to become a well-known brand which people will associate with high quality and good service.

It all sounds very impressive and exciting. Whether people like it or not, veterinary practices in this country are changing, and this could be the future of small-animal practice.

Anyway, after describing the company, he moved on to the specific job, which was going to be in Swansea. It's going to be pretty hard work, starting at 8 a.m. and finishing at 7 p.m. every day, and having to work every other weekend. It'll also mean working solo for the first few months as they only plan initially to have one vet in each surgery, but as the client base builds up, a second vet will be brought in to share the workload.

At the end of the interview, he offered me the job – just like that. I was pretty surprised, to say the least, I thought I'd have to wait a few days or even weeks to find out, but no, he just said, 'So do you want the job then?'

I said that I'd like a few days to think it over and see what Emma thought before committing myself, and he was fine with that. I'm going to let him know at the beginning of next week.

7.00 p.m. Bideford Knackered! I just made it back in time for evening surgery, which was full, of course. Been thinking about the job a lot on the way back and I think I'd be a fool to turn down such a well-paid and exciting job. I hope Emma thinks it's a good idea and doesn't mind me living in Swansea. That's the only real problem, the distance from where Emma will, hopefully, be working. Peter did say that after a year or so it would be quite possible they would be opening a branch in Bristol, so I could move there, which would be miles better.

Friday 15 August

Had a long chat with Emma about the job and things in general and she seems pretty happy for me to take it, although she did say that she was a bit worried about us being so far apart from each other. We looked on the map and it should only take an hour and a half, so we'd be able to see each other quite regularly, if not as much as we do at the moment. The money would be very useful, though, I could help pay off Emma's massive debts from university.

Saturday 16 August

6.15 p.m. M5 services, south of Bristol Just rang Emma to tell her that I've decided not to take the job.

After morning surgery I thought I should at least go and see where I was going to be working if I accepted the job, so I drove off to Swansea to look at the place. It was in a pet superstore called Pets at Home, which was in a characterless industrial estate on the east of the city, flanked by Curry's and The Furniture Warehouse. Pets at Home advertised the presence of its in-store Companion Care veterinary surgery, along with a grooming parlour and a dog and cat re-homing service, on large boards outside the store.

I wandered in and found the surgery at the back of the

store. I explained who I was to the smartly dressed nurse who was at the front desk, and asked if I could have a look around.

'No problem,' she said in a broad Welsh accent, 'just go through. Andre, the vet, is back there somewhere.'

I walked through, past the waiting area, complete with Companion Care promotional video and fish tank, and the two consulting rooms, which opened off the corridor leading into the prep room and kennel area. Everything was very new-looking and organized, and the range of equipment was impressive (blood machine, decent microscope, modern anaesthetic monitors, etc.).

As I moved to look in the operating theatre, which led off the prep room, a tall man of about my age, dressed in a spotless green Companion Care consulting tunic, appeared from the kennels and introduced himself as Andre. He was the vet based in the Cardiff branch, but was also covering the Swansea practice until the new vet started.

I had quite a long chat with him about the job and what it entailed, and left after half an hour or so, less convinced that this was the job for me than I had been when I walked in. It wasn't that I'd seen anything which had made me worry about the standards or equipment levels or anything like that, it was just that I began to have some doubts about how I would cope with working such long hours cooped up in a small surgery with no other vets to talk to or discuss cases with.

On the long drive home, I started to realize quite how far it was between Bristol and Swansea, and the implications of my taking the job on my relationship with Emma. Thirty thousand pounds would be great, but I finally decided that I needed to get my priorities right and put our relationship first. What would be the point in having lots of money if I was left on my own, with no time to spend it and no one to enjoy it with?

Emma was really surprised by my decision, but happy as well.

Now I've just got to tell Companion Care that I don't want their job after all. Oh, yes, and just the little matter of finding another job!

Monday 18 August

10.15 a.m. I was too cowardly to speak to Peter Eville, so I rang up the Companion Care HQ and left a message with the personnel manager saying that due to various reasons I had decided not to accept the job offer. I'm sure that I've done the right thing, and Emma's definitely pleased. We spent a couple of hours on the beach walking the dogs and talking about our future yesterday, and decided that we should make an effort to find jobs which allow us to live together, because living apart like we are at the moment is not helping our relationship. If I'd ended up in Swansea, we'd have only seen each other once or twice a week at most, and I'm not sure that we could have survived that.

The BBC are here again this week, for their final filming session in Bideford. Amanda is directing, because Sarah's still off doing something else. Amanda is excellent, though, and now that I'm getting used to having her asking the questions, I'm finding it just as easy as it was with Sarah. The only problem with Amanda is that every time she asks a question she tries to encourage your reply by smiling at you from behind the camera. Unfortunately the smile tends to turn into a mad-looking grin, which either makes me want to start laughing, or I end up so mesmerized by her insane grimace that I forget to answer her question. I think I'll have to have a word with her about it, I hope she doesn't get offended.

1.30 p.m. Grin sorted (Emma the researcher had a quiet word about behind-the-camera facial expressions, and since then

Amanda's restricted herself to the odd tentative smile and occasional raised eyebrow).

They filmed a good case this morning. Mr Robey, a friendly man of about fifty, brought Trixie, his golden retriever, in for a biopsy. I'd seen him a couple of times over the past month because Trixie has had a progressively worsening discharge from her right nostril which hasn't even responded to long courses of potent antibiotics. Last week when he brought her in, there was a small lump protruding from the end of her nostril, and I noticed that the side of the nose was swollen. I suspected that it might be more than just a nasty infection and could be some form of cancer, so I booked her in to have a biopsy done today.

Under a general anaesthetic, I examined the mass, which appeared to extend from the external opening of the nostril deep into the nose. I had considered trying to remove it when I saw it last week, but now I could appreciate quite how deep it was, I immediately abandoned any ideas of heroic surgery. If there was a chance of removing the mass, it would only be if I referred the case to a more specialized and experienced surgeon.

I took a small sample from the mass and put it in a formalin-filled jar, to be sent to the lab for histo-pathology. Then, while she was unconscious, I took several X-rays to see how far into the nasal cavity the mass extended, and if there was any evidence of spread to the lungs. If it was a nasty tumour, and there were secondaries in the chest, then there would be little hope for her.

Helen developed the films as Trixie recovered in her kennel and I waited anxiously. I really hoped that the mass was small and the lungs were clear. Trixie's a great dog and Mr Robey seems like a nice owner. He's a timid, middle-aged man who obviously adores her.

Helen brought the films up from the darkroom in the cellar and we looked at them together on the viewing screen. The lungs looked fine: there was no evidence of any secondary tumours. The pictures of the nose, however, produced less welcome results. The mass was easily visible and extended deep into the bony tissues of the nasal cavity.

I've spoken to Mr Robey on the phone and told him that what I've found is pretty bad news, and the outlook for Trixie is poor. I did say, however, that if he did want to look into the possibility of removing the mass, then I would talk to Jeff Lane, the specialist ear, nose and throat surgeon who taught me at Bristol. He said, obviously upset by the news, he would try anything if it meant there might be a chance of getting her better again.

3.15 p.m. Finally got through to Jeff Lane at Bristol. Before I could even try to ring him, the BBC spent about half an hour messing around trying to set up some sound recording gear to tape both sides of our conversation. Most of the time they are very good and don't hold things up to much, but occasionally they really get in the way and cause delay. I haven't quite resorted to telling them to go away and leave me in peace, but there's certainly been a few times when I've come very close to snapping!

When I was eventually allowed to use the phone it took another half an hour before I could get through to Jeff, because he was busy on the phone organizing a trip to South America. Because he's got such a good reputation as a surgeon, particularly on horses, he gets paid vast sums of money to go all over the world and operate on valuable horses, and teach other vets how to do new ops.

Anyway, when I did speak to him and described the case, he seemed to think there might be a chance of operating on Trixie and, depending on the results of the biopsy and Mr Robey agreeing, he would see her as soon as possible.

Mr Robey's coming in at five to pick Trixie up, so I'll see what he wants to do. I hope he does go for the referral option, because it would be fantastic if something could be done.

The BBC also would love it if she went to Bristol for treatment. Not only would it be really interesting to see what happens, but it would make a good story to see me referring a case back to my old lecturer for help.

Wednesday 20 August

Trixie's biopsy results are back and show that, as Jeff Lane suspected, the mass is a nasty tumour. I spoke to Mr Robey this morning and told him that although the results had showed the lump was a malignant tumour, there was still a possibility it could be removed. I also said if we did nothing then she would most likely go downhill pretty rapidly and may not survive for more than a few more weeks.

On Monday he said he would probably decide to go for the referral option, and today he said he and his wife had definitely decided that it would be the best thing. So I rang up Bristol again and booked an appointment for this Friday. Now it's up to Jeff.

I did mention the fact that it was going to be pretty expensive, but Mr Robey said that Trixie is insured, so money isn't a problem.

The BBC have gone to film Trixie at home. They are definitely going to follow her progress at Bristol, although after some of the things that happened when they filmed *Vet's School* a couple of years back, I'm not sure quite how welcome they are going to be. There was quite a lot of tension when they were first around, because people were very wary of the cameras, but it was all made an awful lot worse when a very senior member of the clinical staff found a notebook that had been used by the BBC director. Unfortunately, he'd used the book to jot down his personal thoughts on various individuals at the school, and not all of what he'd written was particularly complimentary to the people involved, especially the section written about the person who found the book (tyrannical overbearing old witch were his exact words I think). This caused a major upset and the cameras were almost thrown off the site. In the end they were allowed to stay, but under very tight supervision from the clinical staff.

Thursday 21 August

Still no decent-looking jobs in the *Vet Record*. I think I might do locum work for a month or two until a suitable job comes up near wherever Emma ends up. She's still waiting to hear about the residency at Bristol. I hope she finds out about it soon because if she's not going to get it then she needs to get looking for something else pretty quickly otherwise we're both going to be out on the streets with nowhere to go and no money!

BBC have gone. Amanda was very happy with the filming they did this week, and said they've now got enough for at least three episodes with us in. I asked when they were planning to be shown and she said it would probably be the end of September. Only a month and my life will be broadcast across the nation!

I wonder what it'll be like, seeing myself on telly.

Sunday 24 August

Lovely relaxing last-ever weekend off in Bideford. Emma was off as well so she came up and we did very little except walk the dogs and a bit of surfing (only two feet but offshore and sunny) and grassboarding. The new aluminium prototype, which I picked up on Friday, is fantastic. It's much lighter and works really well.

I've just started to panic slightly because I've realized that in eight days' time I'm leaving, and I've got nowhere to go to! I think I'll move in with Emma while she's still there, but after she leaves her job (early September), unless one of us has found some work we are going to be stuffed! That's the trouble with vet jobs: you usually get a house and car, once you leave you suddenly find yourself homeless and transportless.

I wonder how Trixie got on at Bristol on Friday. I really hope the outcome is good. I also hope I haven't made some horrible mistake in my treatment or diagnosis, and that when Jeff Lane sees her, he doesn't decide it's in fact something completely different to what I've said it is, and if I'd treated it in a different way, she could have been saved. I think that's pretty unlikely, but I worry about it anyway!

Monday 25 August

10.30 a.m. Mr Robey has just rung up and said that, sadly, Jeff Lane had decided that there was nothing that could be done to help Trixie. Apparently when he'd taken detailed X-rays of the nose, he'd seen that the tumour extended so deep into the bones that, in order to remove the tumour, they would have had to remove most of her face. Even if such an operation had been feasible, I'm sure Mr Robey wouldn't have put Trixie through such a traumatic and painful experience.

I rang Jeff Lane, who said that as there was no surgical treatment possible, the only hope was that a high dose of steroids might help to slow down the growth of the tumour and give Trixie a little longer. I asked about other treatments such as radiotherapy or chemotherapy, but he said neither were suitable for this type of tumour (chemotherapy is pretty widely used by many practices in dogs and cats, and even radiotherapy is starting to become more commonly used as well, but only in specialist centres).

So that's that then. I've put her on steroids, with antibiotics to cover her against any infections as the steroids will lower her immune defences. I suspect, however, that it won't be long before Mr Robey will have to decide that the kindest thing would be to put her to sleep. Already she is finding it quite distressing to breathe and has started to have nose-bleeds. I told Mr Robey to keep a close eye on her, and when he and his wife think the time has come, to bring her up and we'll put her out of her misery.

Poor old Trixie, and poor old Mr and Mrs Robey. Still, I suppose the dog is twelve years old, which is a pretty good age for a retriever. It's still upsetting, even though we know we've tried everything and didn't just write her off without making an effort to find out exactly what was wrong with her and see if there were any treatment options available.

Wednesday 27 August

Happier news today. Mrs Powell rang up in an excited rush this morning to say that the eggs have hatched, and to ask if I wanted to come round and see the hatchlings. I said I would be round as soon as I'd finished surgery so, after a fairly quiet morning, I drove round to her bungalow to inspect the new arrivals.

I'd never seen any newly hatched tortoises before, so I didn't really know what to expect. When Mrs Powell lifted the lid of the heated glass tank in which they were now housed, I saw the four new-born tortoises basking under the heat lamp. They were incredible – exactly like their parents only about a twentieth of their size. They were perfect minia-tures, correct in every respect, but only the size of an old fifty-pence piece. Mrs Powell picked one up and offered it some lettuce, which it proceeded to devour with amazing ferocity.

'Wow!' I said, truly impressed. 'They're incredible! So small and delicate.'

'Yes, they are lovely, aren't they?' She agreed, stroking the baby tortoise in her hand. 'Do you want to hold one?'

She held out her hand with the tiny tortoise on and I

gently transferred him to my palm. He looked even more delicate and vulnerable in my big hands, rough from calvings (and grassboarding accidents). Its shell felt hard, but on reading up about tortoises I found it takes several years before it is hard enough to fully protect its occupant from the outside world. I felt so nervous, holding this precious new life in my clumsy hands, that after admiring him for a short time, I placed him back with his siblings on the sand at the bottom of the tank.

'The hatching alarm worked OK then, did it?' I asked, remembering the ingenious contraption that her engineer husband had built for the incubating eggs.

'Oh yes, it was fine. Of course, it was the middle of the night when it went off, but we didn't mind. It was worth it.'

I left after admiring the tortoises for a while longer, and drove back to the surgery thinking sadly that I'd be leaving all these interesting cases and clients behind in under a week. I hope I can come back every now and then to see all the people (and animals) I've enjoyed working with over the last year. I'll miss Ian especially because he's been such a good boss and it's been really fun working with him. I might even miss Keith a little, I mean what am I going to do without someone to drink all the tea and read archaeology books when I'm doing busy surgeries at my new practice (wherever that may end up being)?

Friday 29 August

Very sad day today. Mr Robey rang up this morning and said that Trixie had really gone downhill in the last forty-eight hours and was now in real distress. He and his wife had decided that it was time to let her go, and asked if they could bring her up to the surgery to be put to sleep straight away.

When they arrived I saw what they meant: Trixie was gasping for breath through her narrowed airway, and was constantly swallowing to clear the blood and mucus from her throat. I was shocked at how rapidly she'd deteriorated since I'd last seen her. I'd thought she might be OK for several months at least, rather than just a few days, but I suppose in a way it was better for her to go downhill quickly rather than get worse gradually over a longer time. It made the decision to have her put to sleep much easier for the Robeys, and meant that all of her pain and suffering would come to a much quicker end.

Thankfully the euthanasia went very smoothly and Trixie passed away peacefully. The Robeys were very upset, as expected, but as well as the tears there was also a sense of relief and of a burden being lifted from them. They may have lost their beloved pet, but at least they know now she's not suffering any more. I hope that if I ever end up in a similar state to Trixie, I can go in such a painless, dignified manner and don't have to struggle and suffer to the bitter end.

The Robeys decided that they would like to have Trixie individually cremated and have her ashes back, so I organized that with the cremation service. A sad case to have on my last weekday here but, in a way, I was glad to be there for the Robeys and see the case through to the end.

I'm on call all weekend, then I'm moving on Monday. I'm looking forward to what ever lies ahead, but I'm also getting sadder and sadder about leaving here.

Sunday 31 August

4.00 p.m. Just got back from what may well be my last ever farm call in Bideford. It was a good one to end on, a cow with milk fever right out on the cliffs near Hartland.

I met the farmer, Mr Littlejohn, in the yard of the farm and then we walked out to where the cow was lying, right up against the fence which separated the farm from the cliffs and the sea below. The cow was showing the classic signs of milk fever (recumbent, bent neck, full udder, etc.) and responded quickly when I gave her a bottle of calcium in the vein. While we were waiting for the cow to get up, Mr Littlejohn and I chatted about farming and life in general, looking out over the misty ocean below. We ended up talking about the sea, and he told me that in recent times two people had been killed in sailing accidents on this very stretch of coast beneath his farm. He said that the current was so strong in this area that it can drag you right out to sea, or smash you up on the rocks, and in the past it was notorious for wrecking ships caught in bad winds or tides.

It was really beautiful, leaning against the fence, looking out over the cliffs to the grey sea below. Watching the waves break directly on to sharp-looking rocks lining the foot of the cliff it wasn't hard to imagine how this coast could be treacherous and claim so many lives. Even if you had managed to make it to the shore, there was no way anyone could climb the cliffs to safety. I remembered seeing a chart on the wall of the pub at Hartland Quay which showed the positions of all the shipwrecks in this area and numbers of people killed. It was amazing, every mile or so along the twenty- or thirty-mile stretch of coast had one or two markers indicating a wreck and lives lost.

I am definitely going to miss this place, and especially the sea. There is something special about living next to such a massive, uncontrollable force and having the smell of the sea in the air.

Ah well, I've made my decision.

September

Monday 1 September Last day in Bideford!

12.30 p.m. That was my last ever farm call yesterday, in fact it was the last ever bit of veterinary work that I'll do in the name of Witten Lodge Veterinary Centre. I don't know whether to be happy or sad really. I'm happy that I'm moving on and have got new exciting things to look forward to, but at the same time I'm sad to be leaving such a lovely place and all the people I've got on with so well.

I've just finished loading the van, and now all I have to do is pop into the surgery to pick up the last of my things and I'll be off.

3.00 p.m. Dulverton Well, I've left. It was very emotional, driving away for the last time. I said my final goodbyes to all the nurses and Sue the receptionist, and to Ian and Keith, and promised to return and keep in touch.

I'm now a free man, no work, no being on call. I'm looking forward to relaxing for a week or so. I can't do that for too long, though, because Emma is leaving her job next week, so we need to sort out exactly what we're going to do with our lives.

Saturday 6 September

2.00 p.m. Panic has set in! We've just got back from a night out with Toby and Louise in Bristol and now we've only got about two hours to pack all our stuff into the van we hired in Bristol, clean the house and get out. Emma's replacement, a girl called Imogen, is arriving at 4 p.m! I'd better stop writing and get loading.

4.15 p.m. Just finished loading. The house is a bit of a mess, but we just haven't got time to do any more cleaning up. Also we want to make a quick getaway before Emma's land-lady (fierce Mrs Crook) comes round to check on the place. It's not in too bad a state in general, but a few things have suffered slightly during Emma's time in the house, mainly due to the dogs. They have almost completely devoured one whole armchair and dug a hole in the front wall of the dining room.

No sign of Imogen yet so we're going to leave before either she or Mrs Crook turns up to inspect the house.

6.30 p.m. Tim's house, Bristol I've arranged to stay with Tim in his spare room for a week or two until we get jobs and houses sorted out. Emma's going back to her parents' house in Kent because of the dogs and cats (Tim's allergic to all forms of animal life).

7.40 p.m. Tim's spare room is bulging at the seams. We've piled up all our things and the only space left is a small bit of floor with a mattress on. The room isn't particularly big anyway, but with all of Emma's and my stuff in, it's absolutely packed full. Every time I turn round I knock something off one of the piles – I'm sure that if I toss and turn in my sleep at all I'm going to bring the whole lot down on me and I'll be buried alive!

Emma's just set off for Kent with the animals. I'm going to miss not seeing her, but it'll only be for a week or two. I'm going to try and get some locum work until Emma finds out about the Langford job, which should be very soon.

Tuesday 9 September

I've got some work! I registered with a couple of locum agencies yesterday, and today I was rung up by a vet in Leicester who wants me to go and work for him next week. I don't know much about him, but we're getting pretty short of money so I've accepted anyway.

I've spent the last few days here sorting stuff out and generally getting bored. I almost wish that I was back at work! I thought that having a few weeks off would be excellent – lots of socializing, surf trips and things, but because we're so skint, and all my friends are working, I've ended up sorting out bank stuff, looking for work, and I've even resorted to reading some of my notes from college to refresh my knowledge – a certain sign that I'm bored!

I'm quite looking forward to this locum job next week, it'll be interesting to work at a different place and with new people. I hope it's a decent practice and not some horrible backward place where they use ether for anaesthetics and have only just heard of antibiotics!

Friday 12 September

Emma rang up this afternoon. Apparently the dogs have destroyed the rockery again and are well and truly in her parents' bad books! Apart from dog trouble, she said everything else is fine. The cats are staying with some family friends and have settled in well. (Hopefully they might like them and want to keep them!)

I asked about Penny, Emma's dog, and Emma said she was doing OK, although her back end has started to go from under her more often and she has trouble sitting down. She is fifteen so it's to be expected that she's going to be getting weaker and have more problems, but it's still upsetting for Emma and the rest of the family. I have a feeling that it won't be that long before she may have to be put to sleep.

It must be really hard for Emma, being a vet and knowing that if Penny was a client's dog, she would probably advise the owners that it would be kindest to put her to sleep before too long. Making that decision about the dog she grew up with is going to be so difficult for her. In a way, it would be best for everyone, Penny included, if she passed away peacefully in her sleep.

Sunday 14 September

6.00 p.m. Temple Meads station, Bristol Tim's just dropped me off and I'm about to catch the 6.22 to Leicester. I wasn't quite sure what I was going to need, so I've got a rucksack full of work clothes, a stethoscope and a smelly bag with my waders and calving gown in. I wish that I'd washed them properly after my last farm visit at Bideford – I keep getting funny looks from people when they walk by and smell the festering cow-muck odour emanating from my luggage!

Midnight, Wood Road Veterinary Hospital, Leicester I finally got here at about 10 p.m. after a terrible journey. I had to get a taxi to the practice because Barry Jones, the vet who I spoke to last week, who was supposed to be meeting me, left a message to say he couldn't make it and could I make my own way there.

The practice is right in the middle of a dodgy looking area of the town, with rows of terraced houses and boarded-up shops. The practice itself is two mid-terrace houses knocked together, which has created a large, rambling building with lots of small dark corridors and unexpected steps.

Barry Jones met me when I arrived and showed me round. He seems to be a reasonably nice bloke, if a little odd. He looks like the classic old English eccentric, with wild grey hair and intense eyes, dressed in a tweed jacket and plus fours. I've not really sorted out how many vets work here apart from him, or exactly what he wants me to do, but he said he would give me a proper briefing tomorrow.

The worst thing so far is the accommodation. After he showed me round the practice he took me into the flat, which is on the first floor next door. He said, as we walked in, 'It's not quite finished yet because I only bought it a couple of weeks ago, so you'll have to put up with a few things not working until I get them sorted out later in the week.'

He wasn't exaggerating when he said that it wasn't quite finished – hardly started would have been a better description. There is virtually no furniture, no curtains, no phone, no hot water and a kitchen which would be at home in a grotty student flat.

I'm very glad I brought a sleeping bag, otherwise I would be sleeping on a nasty-looking stained mattress with only a thin yellow blanket for warmth.

I am not looking forward to spending the next ten days in here!

Monday 15 September

7.30 a.m. Not a good night's sleep. First the people in the flat below had loud music on until about 1.30 a.m. and, as soon as that had stopped, a car started racing up and down the street with music blaring out of the open windows. I really don't feel like starting a new job today.

8.45 a.m. Just met Barry and he's given me another tour of the practice, and a bit of a shock. After showing me where most of the drugs and equipment were, he looked at his watch and said, 'Right, you should be fine, I'll see you on Thursday then.'

'What?' I replied, hoping I'd misheard. Surely he couldn't expect me to run his practice without him on my first day.

'I'll see you on Thursday,' he repeated. 'Didn't I say on the phone that one of the reasons I need you here is because I'm going to be away for a couple of days? I'm taking the old girl up to Doncaster for a rally.'

'Old girl?'

'Vintage car. I race vintage cars as a bit of a hobby. I was a professional driver for a few years, but I had to stop because they kept taking my licence away. Anyway, I've got to dash, you should be OK on your own. If you need help, ring

Heather and she'll come in, and you've got Maria here as well.' And with that he rushed out of the front door.

He'd only just introduced me to Maria, a recently qualified Spanish vet who appears to be his only assistant. She seems very friendly, but her English is pretty poor. Barry said she only did the operating at the moment because her English isn't up to consulting work yet.

So now I'm on my own, except for a few nurses and receptionists, and another vet who can't speak English. What a fun week this is turning into!

11.15 a.m. Just finished morning surgery, which was packed. I was really rushed because there were no nurses to help me count tablets or write labels, so between each consultation I had to run out into the dispensary, frantically search for the right drugs, sort the labels out, and take them through to the front desk.

Now I've just been told that I'm already late for the next surgery, which is out at one of the branches about five miles away in a little village.

This is a nightmare!

12.30 p.m. Finished first branch surgery, on my way to number two in the clapped-out old diesel van which is the practice 'Veterinary Ambulance'. It's the worst vehicle I've ever been in. Not only does it feel about as MOT-worthy as a grassboard with an engine, but the passenger footwell is full of empty beer cans and the back is piled up with a random jumble of veterinary equipment.

The branch surgery I've just done was in a small lock-up surgery in a village just outside the town, and now I'm heading right back across town, to what I've been told is the worst part of town, to the next one.

1.20 p.m. Finished branch number two, which turned out to be a grotty little converted shop. The windows at the front are protected by metal mesh and the reinforced glass in the door is partially smashed. Inside is just as bad, with the bare minimum of drugs and equipment in the single consulting room, and a spartan waiting room.

The worst bit, however, is the kennels out the back. Behind the office area are a couple of rooms with a few kennels against the walls. When I walked in, the stench was grim and the kennels themselves are in a foul state, with encrusted faeces covering the metal surfaces. Only one was occupied, with three poor little kittens sharing the worst-smelling cage. They looked terrible, with matted coats and mucky eyes.

I asked the nurse who was doing reception about them, and she said they were strays they were trying to re-home. I asked how long they had been there and if they ever got cleaned out or checked over. She said she didn't really know because she'd only started at the practice last week, but they were being fed by the nurse who lived above the branch.

In the end, I checked them over and started them on some antibiotics for the flu, and asked the nurse to make sure their cage was cleaned out at least once a day.

That's really upset me, seeing those poor animals in such a state. I just hope this is a one off and the practice doesn't let things like this happen regularly.

7.20 p.m. Finally finished, although I'm on call. After a very short lunch break, I had to help Maria with the last couple of ops and then do the two branches which I'd already done this morning again, plus the third branch and then the main surgery again. The third branch is in a pet superstore in a retail park on the edge of town, very similar to the Companion Care surgeries. Although I found it quite strange working inside a large superstore, it's the best of the branches because it's relatively clean and well equipped. The nurse working there, called Rhona, is also the only one I've met so far who seems to have any clue as to what she's doing. None of the others are qualified nurses, and most of them seem to have only been at the practice for a few weeks.

I'm absolutely knackered now, after a bad night's sleep and doing seven surgeries in one hectic day. I can't see how this place keeps going, it's so disorganized and chaotic and understaffed.

I really wish I could just pack my bag and leave. The last thing I want to do is spend another night in this horrible flat, with the prospect of nine more days working in this place.

I'd give anything to swap this for another week working in Bideford – doing too many morning surgeries is nothing compared to doing seven different surgeries in one day, especially in such a terrible place!

Tuesday 16 September

7.45 a.m. Oh no! I really am here, and I've got to face a seven-surgery day again. A better night's sleep, but only just (the people downstairs finished their party at 1.15 a.m., and thankfully the boy-racers didn't return).

10.30 a.m. Busy morning again. I saw a couple of worrying cases, two animals in for post-op checks which had nasty discharging wounds. One of them was an English bull terrier which had had an exploratory operation done last week, and now the abdominal wound was open and oozing nasty-looking pus. The other was a spaniel which was castrated a week ago and now had a nasty infected wound, a bit like the one I treated in Bideford, although not quite as bad.

I got them both on to strong antibiotics and asked them to come back in a couple of days. It doesn't say much for the standard of operating at the practice if this kind of post-op problem is happening on a regular basis.

I told Maria about them and she looked on the cards to see who had operated on them and, to my surprise, both ops had been done by Barry. I suppose I'd immediately assumed that Maria must have been responsible because she appeared to do most of the operating and was less experienced than Barry.

Maybe it was a coincidence, all vets occasionally get problems like these, although it has to be said that to get two together that are so bad is pretty worrying.

2.15 p.m. On my way to the superstore surgery, no lunch, very bad mood, wish I wasn't here.

7.50 p.m. Just had a long talk with Emma on the phone and poured out my woes to her. I told her that I was very close to leaving. It's not the hard work, I can put up with that, it's the state of the practice (and the flat).

I've never seen a practice as badly run as this one, and worse than that is the way the animals and clients are treated as a result. I end up having to ferry animals around in the back of the van to bring them back to the main surgery for operations, and then they are quite often forgotten about or misplaced or sent to the wrong surgery after their ops – it's a real mess! The standard of treatment is pretty worrying as well. I saw a couple more infected wounds this afternoon, and quite a few cases with obvious problems which had gone unnoticed and untreated.

For example, a lady brought in an elderly Labrador with a non-healing wound on its back where it had been bitten some weeks previously. As soon as I looked at it I thought to myself: This dog has Cushing's syndrome, because it was showing classic symptoms – a large pot belly, hair loss and thin skin. When I questioned the owner, I found out that it was also drinking excessively and weeing all over the house – two more important symptoms of the disease. From the record card I could see that this problem had been ignored, and Barry had just been trying to get the wound to heal using antibiotics. If the dog did indeed have Cushing's syndrome then there was little chance of the wound healing until the disease was treated, as another of the effects of the syndrome

257

is poor wound healing. I've taken an initial blood sample to see if there is evidence of Cushing's and if there is, I'll talk to the owner about further tests and treatment.

It really amazed me that Barry had missed such a clear-cut case as this. It's not as if I'm a supervet who has picked up a very early case of an obscure disease, it's an obvious case of a relatively common disorder which would be diagnosed by most vets as soon as the animal walked in the consulting-room door.

This really is turning into one of the worst weeks of my life – I'm stuck in this horrible flat, working at the most disorganized, badly run practice in the world.

I am counting the hours to next Tuesday when I can leave this terrible place!

11.55 p.m. Had to see a dog with a cut foot at the surgery. I tried to get hold of a nurse to give me a hand, but the flat above the practice where I thought there would be an on-duty nurse was empty. Because this is an accredited Veterinary Hospital, there should be a qualified nurse on duty at all times. As there aren't even any fully qualified nurses working at the practice, it was asking a bit much to expect there to be one on call, I suppose, but then it shouldn't be called a Veterinary Hospital if it doesn't conform to the required standards.

In the end I managed to sort the dog out on my own, but it's pretty bad that a place advertising itself as a hospital practice hasn't even got a nurse, qualified or not, on duty overnight.

12.42 a.m. No! The bloody boy-racers are back!

1.50 a.m. As I've been lying awake, listening to the bass line of some very loud music pumping out of the open windows of the black XR3i which is doing wheel spins outside my window, I've finally worked out what's going on. It's obviously because I was bad to Blackie the devil cat in Bideford and now he's got his revenge by sending me to veterinary hell!

If this is what lies in store for me in the afterlife as an unloving cat owner, I'm going to start a cat sanctuary and spend all my money on fluffy cat beds and toy mice – anything to avoid eternity here!

Wednesday 17 September

1.30 p.m. Slightly quieter this morning because one of the branches was cancelled due to not enough staff. As a result I stayed here for most of the morning and helped Maria with the ops.

I can now see why so many of the animals are getting post-op infections. The operating theatre is very cramped and dirty, and the instruments and drapes are poorly sterilized. The theatre is a tiny partitioned area of the prep room, with barely enough space to move, let alone operate satisfactorily. As well as the cramped room, the operating table is old and dirty, and the instruments are routinely used for several ops between being sterilized. Everything is disorganized, as I've come to expect here, and, as a result, it is nearly impossible to operate effectively and to maintain any semblance of sterility.

The nurse who was in charge of the anaesthetic was very friendly and helpful, but as she was only sixteen and had started just a month earlier, she knew very little about monitoring anaesthetics in particular or nursing in general. That made the operations even more risky, and I was pretty surprised that both the dogs I operated on actually survived. Whether they succumb to post-op infection is another matter. I loaded them up with antibiotics to try and stop infection taking hold, but I wouldn't be at all surprised if they do get wound infections, considering quite how unsterile the operations were.

I had a long chat with Maria while we were operating

(her English is certainly up to conversation, so I can't really see why Barry doesn't let her consult) about the practice and how bad it was here.

She completely agreed with me and said that the only reason she was working here was because there are so few jobs in Spain that she needed to take whatever she could get. She also said that most vets in this country were pretty unwilling to take on foreign vets, especially if their English wasn't perfect, so she was grateful to have found a job at all, even if it wasn't great and the pay was terrible.

I suspect that a lot of foreign vets like Maria get really exploited in jobs like these, where they get worked really hard and are paid a pittance. Part of the reason is that the training vets get in some countries is much poorer than in this country, especially when it comes to actual experience of consulting and operating. In England, all vet students have to spend about six months seeing practice with vets during the final three years of training, and that's where most of the practical skills of consulting and surgery are learnt. On many foreign courses, vets can qualify having never done a cat spay or dog castration, and are expected to take low-paid, or even unpaid, jobs to gain that experience when they first leave college. As a result, there is the potential for unscrupulous practice owners to exploit the situation and take advantage of the willingness of these newly qualified vets to work for minimal wages in order to gain the experience that they should have got at college.

Damn! I've just spent the entire twenty minutes that I had for lunch waffling on in my diary, so now I'm going to have to eat my lovely looking dried-up sausage roll while piloting the chariot of doom over to the terrible branch number two. I hope the kittens have been cleaned out today, because they were still in a right state yesterday. Poor things, I bet they wish they'd never been rescued and had been left to take their chances with the world on their own.

3.10 p.m. That place gets worse. The kittens' cage was as grim as ever, and just to add to the general ambience of the place, there was the body of a dog that had been put to sleep yesterday lying on the floor in the kennel room. It was a big Labrador which I'd put to sleep because of bad back legs, and it was supposed to have been taken back to the main surgery last night to be put in the freezer, but it had been forgotten. As a result I had to load the body up into the van and carry it around all afternoon as I went to the other branches, before I could take it back to the main surgery.

8.10 p.m. Three days down, six to go. At least Barry is back tomorrow so I shouldn't be quite so rushed.

I'm off to find an Indian takeaway. I think I deserve a treat.

9.00 p.m. Not an Indian takeaway to be found for love nor money. All the shops are either boarded up or covered with heavy-duty metal shutters. In the end I had to resort to a very dodgy looking pasty and chips from the only place that was open within about a mile of the practice. This place just gets worse and worse!

9.20 p.m. Emma, the researcher from the BBC, has just rung to ask if they can come and film me here for a couple of days. I warned them about the state of the place, but they seemed to think that it would be quite interesting, so I said I'd ask Barry when he gets back tomorrow. I really hope they can come, because some friendly company would be great.

I also rang Emma again and begged her to come down at the weekend. It would be so much more bearable if she was around. She said she would try.

Friday 19 September

Yesterday was slightly better than the beginning of the week. Barry came back yesterday morning, but I didn't really see much of him until evening surgery because he was doing large-animal visits. He seemed quite agitated and stressed when he finally returned to the practice, and other than a few enquiries about how things had gone while he'd been away, he hardly spoke at all.

Today things reached an all time low. It has been a disaster from start to finish, even by the standards of this place. Firstly there was confusion about who was doing the different surgeries, which ended up with me doing them all, and then I had the horrifying experience of seeing Barry operate and the end results of some of his operations. I realize that not all vets do things to the same standards and some vets are better at surgery than others, but what I've seen this morning was just awful.

Firstly, he proudly showed me the X-rays of a dog whose leg he'd repaired the week before. The pre-op film showed the dog's femur smashed into five or six sharp fragments. The X-ray taken after the repair showed the fragments still in roughly the same disorganized array, but with several metal pins going through the leg attached to two external bars. It looked to me as if there would be absolutely no way the leg would heal, with the bone fragments so badly aligned, but Barry seemed confident enough.

'The thing to remember with fractures like this is that as long as the pieces are roughly in the right place, and you stick the dog in a cage for a month, it'll be fine,' he explained in the stern, authoritative manner which seems to be his normal mode when talking to me or Maria. He obviously belonged to the very old-fashioned school of thought which said that as long as an animal can't move too far, any broken bones will heal.

The dog came in shortly afterwards for a check-up, and Barry ended up admitting it to be hospitalized because the owners weren't happy keeping it confined in a cage at home. The dog is a lovely little Jack Russell terrier called Barney, and he really doesn't look well. The external fixator on his leg is holding the fragments in place, but I still can't see how they are going to heal if they aren't even in line, let alone being compressed together. He looks very depressed and the leg is obviously extremely painful even though he's on some powerful painkillers.

Worse was to come, however. As Maria was having a well-earned day off, Barry and I did the operating between us after morning surgery. I did a couple of spays while Barry was sorting out Barney and, as I was finishing the last spay, he started the final op, which was a dog castration. I was using the operating theatre but instead of waiting five minutes for me to finish, he went ahead with the operation in the prep room, or rather the small grotty area the other side of a partition from the theatre. I watched him through the glass in the partition and was horrified to see how he did what should be a simple and safe operation.

He knocked the dog out with thiopentone in the vein but then, instead of intubating the dog and putting it on gas to give a good, safe and controlled anaesthetic, he just taped the syringe into the dog's leg and topped up the injection every time the dog showed signs of waking up.

Once it was vaguely asleep, he gave his hands a cursory wash and started to do the operation without even tying the dog's legs out of the way, let alone clipping and scrubbing the operation site. Throughout the rushed procedure he was using his hands to move the legs out of the way and top up the anaesthetic, so any semblance even of cleanliness (sterility was a non-starter) was abandoned. Not only was the operation performed with no attempt at sterility and with an extremely unsafe anaesthetic, but even the technique he used to do the actual castration was awful. Instead of careful ligation of the blood vessels and cords, he simply tied the cords in a knot in the same manner that a cat castration is done. This works in cats because they are small and the blood vessels are easy to tie off in this manner, but in a dog, unless the vessels are tied off properly with suture material, there is a very real risk that they will bleed – a complication which can be life-threatening. Towards the end of the operation, which only took about five or six minutes instead of the more usual fifteen to twenty, the dog was waking up (the syringe of thiopentone was empty by this point), so he was desperately trying to hold the dog on the table while suturing the wound closed. In the end he just about managed to cobble it together before the dog leapt from the table in obvious distress.

It really was the worst piece of surgery I've ever seen and if that's how he operates normally, then I'm surprised anything ever leaves this place alive.

When I got back a couple of hours later I found Maria desperately operating on the dog again.

I'd had to go and do the branch surgeries while Barry went out to a couple of large-animal calls, so the dog was left alone in the kennel until Maria came in on the off-chance to check on one of her in-patients. She found the poor dog that Barry had castrated semi-conscious in a massive pool of blood. She'd immediately put it on a drip and tried to staunch the flow of blood from the wound, but with little success. The artery to the testicle comes directly off the aorta so when it bleeds, it really bleeds.

By the time I returned, Maria had managed to stabilize the dog and had just anaesthetized it again in order to try and locate the bleeding vessel and tie it off properly. I scrubbed up to help, but even with the two of us operating, it took about half an hour before we were both happy that the bleeding was under control.

Instead of a quick, relatively painless operation after which the dog would have gone home the same night, it ended up having two operations, losing several pints of blood and having to stay in overnight.

I heard Barry explaining to the owners how there had been a minor complication with the operation, and that we were keeping him in overnight as a precaution. I felt like ringing them back and saying, 'Your dog nearly died because of the incompetence of the vet who operated on him.' But of course I didn't. Vets aren't supposed to criticize each other publicly, for fear of bringing the profession into disrepute, so I'm taking out my frustration and anger in this diary. Times like these make me really question rules like that – the public have a right to know what goes on, and if their animals are being treated well or not.

I thought about telling the Royal College about what I've seen here this week, but I remember being told by someone that the Royal College is run by partners, for the benefit of partners, and assistants like me have very little influence. In a situation like this, it would be my word against his and they would accept his. Also, apparently, if you make an allegation of bad practice, you are labelled a trouble-maker from then on.

Bloody inbred political crap!

The only good news from today is that Emma is coming down tomorrow, and the BBC are arriving on Monday. Barry wasn't overly keen on them filming, he kept on about the media controlling people's lives and stuff, but in the end he said that as long as he had some control over what they shot, he'd put up with them.

Sunday 21 September

Emma turned up yesterday lunchtime, which was such a relief. It's been one of the worst weeks of my life, not just the job, but the flat as well. Having Emma here will make things better, and I've only got two more days left in this hell hole, so hopefully I'll survive.

I told Emma all about the job and she was pretty shocked. I said how I thought that the public should have an idea of what goes on behind the scenes at their vet's, and that vets should be much more accountable to the public, and people should get much more information about their vet practice and how it compares to others.

I reckon a register of practices would be a good idea. It could have details of the vets (and nurses) who work in each practice, the equipment, types of operations carried out, how much the fees are, and reports from qualified inspectors. Routine inspections are essential, I think, to ensure that practices like this one can't exist, because at present most practices are never checked to see that they are up to any kind of standard. Only practices which apply to become veterinary hospitals are inspected, and if this place can get away with passing the inspection and call itself a hospital, then something is going very wrong somewhere.

Veterinary hospitals are supposed to be top-quality practices which offer twenty-four-hour hospitalization facilities, with qualified nurses on the site at all times to look after in-patients through the night. Only practices which have passed the (supposedly) rigorous inspection, and paid their fee, are allowed to call themselves a hospital and advertise as such. Quite how Wood Road passed that test I have no idea. Twenty-four-hour hospitalization facilities here involve the animal being put in a room marked 'Intensive Care' and left there from 7 p.m. until 8.30 the next morning. The nearest qualified nurse is probably several miles away in a different practice.

Not only is the intensive care hospitalization a joke (not if you're the patient), but Barry has the gall to charge the owners £35 per night for the privilege of having their animal put in a cage in a room overnight.

The worrying fact is that he gets away with it and his clients never know. If an animal were to die in the middle of the night while in his intensive care facility, he could tell the owner how despite their valiant efforts to resuscitate poor little Rover, he passed away in the nurse's arms in the early hours, and they would never know the difference. As long as the only way that people can judge their vet is by how they come across in the consulting room, bad vets can get away with this kind of abuse of trust.

I hope and suppose that places like this are very rare, and that 99 per cent of vets don't operate like this, but things need to change. It may only be a tiny proportion of practices which are as bad as this, but that's no consolation to the animals and clients who suffer as a result.

Monday 22 September

8.30 a.m. Amanda and Emma from the BBC, along with Steve the cameraman and a soundman called John, have just turned up. I really hope they get some good evidence on film of how bad this place is so that the public can see how terrible it is. I suppose they probably wouldn't show anything too bad for fear of being sued, but they might be able to portray the overall badness of the place!

9.45 a.m. BBC gone! Barry had a massive row with Amanda about who had control over what was filmed. He wanted Amanda to sign a form he'd written saying that he had absolute editorial control over what was filmed, and that they had to ask his specific permission to film anything. There was no way Amanda could agree to that because they have to be able to decide what they want to film and what they want to show in the finished programmes. When they've filmed before, they've always completely respected the decision of the client if they didn't want to be included, or if I didn't want them to film a certain case for whatever reason. Also, when they've finished editing the films, they always show us and change any bits that we're not happy with.

Barry just wanted complete control over what they did, which was never going to work, so after a few minutes they decided that there was no point arguing with him and they left. I was really sorry to see them go, it would have been good to have some friendly faces in the practice. I think Barry was being much too overprotective about what they could film in his practice – it's not like they want to make a serious investigative documentary about it, they just want a few non-controversial cuddly animal stories!

12.45 p.m. Amanda has just rung me and apologized for deserting me. She said that even though they weren't there for very long, they still thought it was a terrible place, and they were tempted to rescue me by whisking me off with them! It would be lovely just to get up and leave, but I've only got one more day left, and Emma and I really need the money, so I'm going to grit my teeth and bear it for one more day.

Castration dog finally went home after a weekend of 'intensive care'. It was lucky to be alive.

11.30 p.m. On my own in the flat again as Emma had to go back this evening. She still hasn't heard about the job at Langford, so it's really hard for us to make any definite plans about what we are going to do, or where we're going to live. I'm going back to Tim's tomorrow after I get out on parole from this place, and start looking for a job around Bristol, on the assumption that Emma either gets the Langford job, or she gets another job in the same area. The one thing we've definitely decided is that we want to live together, so we need jobs which are close together.

Tuesday 23 September

8.00 a.m. Last day!!!

1.15 p.m. Only six hours to go! This morning wasn't too bad. I did a horse visit, which made a bit of a change. It was only a routine vaccination, but it was still good to get out of the surgery and see a bit of the countryside.

7.20 p.m. Finished!! I feel as though I've been let out of prison after twenty years inside for a crime I didn't commit.

I had quite a long chat with Barry this afternoon, about all sorts of stuff, including the state of the veterinary profession. He seemed quite surprised that I'd not heard of him before, because apparently he's quite a well-known figure in veterinary politics. He ended up lecturing me for quite a while about how all the changes going on in the profession at the moment are ruining it, especially these new American companies like Companion Care (I didn't mention the fact that I nearly took a job with them). He thinks that once big companies take over vet practices they will start telling their vets how to treat animals and what they can and can't do. Much as I didn't want to agree with him about anything, I had to admit that he had a fair point.

He also told me quite a lot about his chequered past. He left college and went into practice somewhere, but then got bored, so he started racing vintage cars instead. Then he got into some trouble with the Royal College and decided to stop being a vet for a while (or was it decided for him I wonder?) and became a professional racing driver. He did this for a year or two before the racing authorities took away his licence for some reason, and he was forced back into vetting. He came to this practice as a locum, like me, but ended up buying it and has been here ever since.

He's obviously a really strong-willed person, convinced that he's right about everything and very unwilling to back down. This has got him into trouble with most forms of authority over the years, including the Royal College, the Racing Drivers Association and, of course, the police. He went on at great length about how the local police were always on his back for a variety of alleged offences ranging from not insuring the practice vans to driving while disqualified (he was innocent of everything, of course, pure unprovoked police harassment).

He's a classic example of a vet who should have been

something else, in his case a racing driver or a politician or something. There are definitely a lot of vets around who become vets for the wrong reasons and then end up not being very good vets or, as in his case, being very bad ones. Some people go into it because they are really clever at school and know that being a vet is supposedly the hardest course to get on. They become a vet because it is a challenge, and don't stop along the way to consider if it's what they really want to do.

I think the fact that it is so hard to get in to vet school is partly to blame – only people with top A-level results stand a chance of getting in, and academic people often don't make the best vets. Good vets have to be pretty clever, but they also need manual skills and a real desire to do the job.

I should include myself in this because, although I mostly love being a vet, there are definitely times when I do wonder if I've chosen the right career. I'm not sure what else I would have done and I have no regrets about doing it, it's just that maybe me being on the course prevented someone else, with a real burning passion to be a vet, from getting on and becoming a better vet.

Emma, for example, wanted to be a vet from the age of about five and has never considered doing anything else. Even when her teachers at school told her that she'd never make it and to try for something less ambitious, she persevered.

It is a strange position to be in because, in a way, having the qualification traps you into doing the one job for the rest of your career. After spending five years and a lot of the taxpayers' money on the training, it's very hard to consider not being a vet at the end of it. Some people do finish the course and decide that it's not for them, but most people practise for a few years at least before thinking about changing careers. I don't know if I'll last the distance and still be a vet when I'm sixty, but I hope that if I do do something else I'll always keep on vetting, even if only part time.

On the other hand, I sincerely hope that Barry isn't still vetting next week, let alone when he's sixty!

9.00 p.m. Tim's house, Bristol Hooray! I'm a free man again! Going down the pub with Tim for a very well-earned pint!

Sunday 28 September

Just about recovered from my week in Leicester. I spent the last few days working on the grassboard because I've been neglecting it recently. I've also been spurred into action by finding a rival board on the internet (Tim's got a computer). At first I thought it was identical to mine and that all my development and effort were going to have been in vain, but as I looked at it more closely, I saw that instead of trying to simulate a snowboard like my board does, this one is just an overgrown skateboard, with a solid deck and no proper bindings. Still, the fact that there is a rival out there is worrying enough, so I've decided to try and really push on with the development and get my board into production asap.

October

Wednesday 1 October

Good news and very bad news. The good news is that I've found out about the first UK grassboarding championships, which are being held in Brighton next weekend.

The bad news is that Emma didn't get the Langford job. She rang up this morning and told me she'd got a letter today which said, 'Due to the high standard of applicants for this position, we are unable to offer you an interview.'

I couldn't believe it! The lecturer who told her to apply in the first place seemed convinced she would get the job, and she only applied because of what he said. She thought all along that she was probably too young and inexperienced, but was convinced by him that she would probably get the position. Now it turns out she hasn't even got an interview, we've wasted two months waiting to hear, and she's had her hopes built up and then dashed.

She didn't actually seem that upset, which surprised me, because I thought she'd really set her sights on it, but she said that in the end she was quite relieved not to get the job because, although it would have been really interesting and good experience, it would have meant three years of low pay and being stuck in one job.

Now at least we can stop waiting and get on with finding a job each!

The grassboarding thing sounds like the perfect opportunity to compare my board with this American rival, which is what everyone will be using at Brighton. I just hope mine is better, because if it turns out someone else has got in there before me and developed a better board, I will be so pissed off. I'm banking on the grassboard to make my millions!

It Really Does Happen To a Vet

Sunday 5 October

8.45 p.m. Emma's parents' house, Kent Excellent weekend, especially today. I came up from Bristol on Friday and we spent yesterday looking for jobs in the *Vet Record* and generally enjoying being together again. Today we went to the grassboarding championships in Brighton, which were fantastic. The BBC came along and filmed it as well, because they're following the story of the grassboard.

The event was organized by the company who are importing the rival 'MBS' grassboard, and was held in Stanmer Park, just outside Brighton. I was pretty nervous on the way down, thinking what I would do if their board turned out to be better than mine, but as soon as we arrived and saw people riding the MBS boards, I knew I was OK. The MBS boards look quite like my board in that they are about the same size and have four wheels, but that's where the similarities end. Whereas my board is flexible and turns due to the bend and tilt of the deck much like a snowboard, the MBS works just like a skateboard. It consists of a solid metal chassis with a wooden deck on top which can't flex at all and steering mechanisms at each end that turn the axles when the board is leant over. Unlike my rubber bush arrangement, the lean on the MBS is controlled via springs – a method I tried and discarded ages ago!

They also just rely on little toe straps to keep you on the board, whereas I use proper snowboard boots and bindings, which hold you firmly in place. Everyone who looked at my board to begin with thought I was mad, strapping myself in so I couldn't get off, but as soon as I'd done a few runs they could see that being strapped in gave me much more control and loads more potential for decent jumps. People also thought it must be much more dangerous, but whenever I fell over on my board, the weight of it just stopped me and I was usually pretty unscathed. People riding the MBS, on the other hand, were having some disastrous bust-ups. The worst ones were where they tried to bale out at speed, but got half-caught in the toe straps and ended up bouncing down the hill with the board semi-attached to one foot, bashing into them as they tried desperately to get free. Luckily the St John's Ambulance was on standby because there were two or three people with quite nasty injuries!

Most of the event was just for people to try out the MBS board, but there were a couple of competitions. I didn't enter the slalom because I wasn't too happy with the tight turning ability of my board (I think it needs some minor modifications to improve it in that department), but I entered the border-cross. This was basically a free-for-all race down a course with some obstacles to negotiate on the way and a small jump at the end. It was really just a bit of fun, not taken too seriously, but I still managed to come second, which wasn't too bad considering I was on my own home-made board and up against people who'd been riding the MBS for quite a while.

I was really happy with the way things went, and I think most of the people there were pretty impressed with my board. It's definitely given me new determination to go ahead and get my board into production.

In fact, Emma and me had a long talk on the way home afterwards about what we should do with our lives and we made a few big decisions. Emma's going to apply for a job that she's seen advertised in Cheltenham, and I'm going to try and find some regular part-time or locum work so that I have some time off to spend working on the grassboard. I think we should be able to earn enough money, and I really feel that I've got to at least try and get the board on the market, otherwise I'll always wonder about what could have been. If someone else comes along with a board like mine and makes a fortune out of it, while I'm plodding along in a full-time job because I was too scared to take the plunge and go for it, I'll be very annoyed, to say the least!

I'm not giving up being a vet, because I do really enjoy

it and I want to keep on doing it. It's more like I'm trying to achieve the best of both worlds – being a successful vet and starting a successful new business.

Now all I've got to do is find a suitable well-paid, good-quality job near Cheltenham and we'll be sorted – assuming Emma likes the job in Cheltenham, and gets it, that is.

Both of us are really getting fed up with all this uncertainty at the moment.

Monday 6 October

Back in Bristol. Emma's gone up for her interview in Cheltenham today. It sounds like a really good practice, but you never know until you see it, I mean Wood Road Veterinary Hospital didn't sound too bad!

The other news is that Emma's sister, Jo, rang up and suggested that we go out and stay with her for a week, as we've got all this time off. The only slight snag is that she lives in Canada, but Emma would love to go because she's not seen her for nearly two years, and I'd really like to meet her. We're going to see how much the flights cost and then see if we can scrape the money together. If we don't go now, we'll never get round to it because we'll be working again.

Friday 10 October

Fantastic news on all fronts! Emma's got the Cheltenham job, we're going to Canada, and I've managed to land a 360° jump on the grassboard!

After the interview on Monday she came down to Bristol for the night before going back to Kent the next day, and was full of enthusiasm for the job. Apparently the place is really nice, the boss is really nice and the town is really nice! The job does sound good, a one in eight out-of-hours rota (because they share the duties with three other local practices), really good facilities, and an enthusiastic boss. The only down side is that the pay isn't wonderful, but according to Emma, it should go up quickly if she gets on well.

She decided she would definitely take the job if she was offered it, and then on Thursday the boss (Barry MacDonald) rang her in Kent and did just that! She starts at the beginning of November, which is just about soon enough to save us from having to resort to eating Pan and Badger as we run out of money!

We've also managed to sort out some cheapish tickets to go to Canada before Emma starts her new job. It's using our last reserves of money, but I can't see when else we'll get the time to go. It's important to Emma, so it's worth the sacrifice of not eating for a few weeks! We fly out a week on Saturday. I'm quite excited, because I've never been to America or Canada before, so it'll be interesting to see what it's like. It'll be good to meet Emma's sister as well. I've met her two younger sisters and get on with them pretty well, but I've only ever seen photos of Jo and spoken to her a couple of times on the phone.

Wednesday 15 October

Frustrating week, because I haven't been able to do much (no money, raining – so no grassboarding – flat surf, no Emma). No part-time jobs in the *Vet Record* within 100 miles of Cheltenham.

Never mind, we're off to sunny Canada in three days! Well, hopefully, snowy Canada – you never know, we might even get some snowboarding in if we're lucky.

Saturday 18 October

8.55 a.m. Gatwick We're off! It's going to be great to get away and have a break from the uncertainty and stress of things here for a week. Even though Emma's got a job, we've still not found anywhere to live (her job doesn't come with a house), and I still haven't got a job. Tim's starting to wish he'd never let us stay, I think, because the room is packed full of our stuff, and he can't look for a permanent tenant until we go. He and Nicky are pretty poor at the moment because they're both changing jobs, so they need the income from a lodger to get by. We've been paying them what they normally get for the room (not even a little reduction for a mate, the tight-fisted so and so!), but I think they want us out fairly soon so they can get someone more settled in.

Anyway, a week away to forget all these problems is going to be superb!

Monday 27 October

Back to reality again. We've had a great time, spent too much money, which we haven't got, but relaxed and forgot about all our house/job woes.

Jo's really nice, and so is her husband Jeff and their son Richard, who's six. We spent the week doing very little, just lazing around, walking their dog (a really nice cross-breed called Chester) and drinking too much (something that seems to be a recurrent theme in our holidays).

We did manage to do a little bit of snowboarding, but it was only on a small hill behind their house because none of the resorts were open.

We ended up buying a snowboard and boots each because they're so much cheaper over there than in this country. A pretty decent board with boots and bindings was about £250, whereas here it'd be about £500. We thought that we'd be saving ourselves money in the long run, so we got the Visa cards out! I think we're going to regret it now we're back and we've got to pay off the bills, but never mind – it's only money!

We're going up to Cheltenham to look for a house to rent on Thursday, but I don't think there's any way we'll have found somewhere by the time Emma starts her job next

Monday. We'll have to stay at Tim's for a bit longer and she can commute for a week or two.

Wednesday 29 October

Things are starting to get better at last. I've got an interview at a practice in Birmingham to do weekend work. It sounds like you have to work pretty hard, but the pay is excellent, and we really need to get some money. I rang up this afternoon and I'm going up there tomorrow for an interview.

If it works out, I can do one or two weekends a month there, and find a job nearer to Cheltenham where I can work two or three days a week. That should bring in enough money and leave me a bit of time to get the grassboard going.

Thursday 30 October

4.15 p.m. I've got a job at last! I'm having a trial weekend on 8/9 November, and if I get on OK, then I should be able to do at least two a month.

The practice seems really busy and a far cry from either Devon or, thankfully, Leicester. It's called Manor Veterinary Centre, and is in a suburb on the west of Birmingham called Halesowen. The practice is in a row of shops on a busy main road and doesn't look particularly impressive from the outside. The name is displayed on a large banner above the shop-front windows of the waiting room, but otherwise it's indistinguishable from the shops on either side. I arrived at about midday, and the waiting room was packed with owners and animals. Three consulting rooms were in use, with a steady flow of patients being called in through each door.

I approached the reception desk, which took up a corner of the waiting room, and told one of the busy receptionists that I was here for an interview. She replied in a thick Brummie accent that they were running a little behind schedule and would I mind waiting a few minutes. I sat down, but didn't have to wait long before one of the vets, a tall man with short grey hair, introduced himself as Paul, one of the partners.

'Follow me, I'll give you a quick guided tour and then we'll go upstairs and have a chat,' he said, taking me through into the office, which lay behind the reception desk.

He showed me around the practice, and I was really impressed with what I saw. It wasn't enormous, but everything was well laid out. The operating theatre was in use, with a shorter, dark-haired vet of about the same age (early thirties) operating on a dog. He introduced himself as Darren, also a partner, and said he'd come and join us upstairs once he'd finished.

It was so nice to see a decent, well-run practice after the shock of Wood Road. There seemed to be qualified nurses everywhere, and the whole place oozed organization and quality (whereas Wood Road had oozed grime and chaos).

After the tour, we went upstairs and sat down in an impressive vets' room with a library of textbooks on one wall and a large conference table in the middle. Darren came in soon after, and then the third partner, an older woman called Mrs MacNauton (no question of first name terms, not that she was unpleasant, far from it, but she had the slightly scary air of a stern mother who one doesn't dare disobey).

They asked me a few questions about what I'd done in Bideford, and what I'd been doing over the last few months, and then explained what the situation was regarding the weekend work.

Basically, a few months ago, they had decided that as partners, they wanted to have more time off at the weekends, but they could also see that weekends could be a very profitable time for the practice to open. Most practices run a Saturday morning surgery, but after that it's just emergencies until Monday. They reasoned that people have most time to come to the vet at weekends, so it was stupid not to be open.

They decided to open all day on Saturday and Sunday, with normal consulting hours and no extra charges, and get part-time vets in to do the work. In the first few months since they started up the weekend opening, it'd been really successful, so now they were looking to expand the weekend workforce – which is where I would come in.

The work does sound pretty hard – consulting all day Saturday and Sunday, and being on call one night (which means staying in the practice flat).

November

Saturday 8 November

8.15 p.m. Manor Vet Centre, Halesowen I'm sitting in the flat above the practice after one of the hardest days of veterinary work I've ever had to do! I arrived at about 8.30 a.m. after leaving Tim's house at about 7 a.m. and met Darren, who worked this morning, and Brian, the other weekend vet on this weekend. Morning surgery started at 9.00, and from then until about 12.15 it was solidly booked; we each saw one client every ten minutes. It took me a while to get used to using a computer for the clients' records and bills, because in Bideford and Leicester all the histories were written by hand on cards. After an hour or so, though, I was beginning to get the hang of it and by the end of the morning I was finding it quite easy, and much better than struggling with dog-eared cards. The main advantages of the computer seem to be never losing the cards (which was always happening in Bideford), and ease of printing out bills and forms.

The practice is so well organized, and I was amazed at how efficient everything was. For example, in Bideford I used to see the clients, write their card, walk through to the dispensary, count out the tablets, write a label and finally take it through to the front desk and the waiting client. The whole process took about half of the allotted consulting time, which meant that either the surgeries would run over time, or I'd have to cut short the consultations. Here, on the other hand, I type the history and treatment into the computer, which automatically prints out the relevant labels in the dispensary, where the nurses dispense the drugs and take them through to the desk. It means that I was able to consult all morning and see about twenty people without having to leave the consulting room (except for occasional tea and wee breaks).

Although it was really hard work, because everything runs so smoothly and efficiently it was much more enjoyable and satisfying than the consulting I used to do in Bideford.

287

The clients seemed really nice and friendly – and I got my first official public recognition!! An elderly lady with a Jack Russell (clip claws and express anal glands) said, 'Ooh, I saw you on telly last night, didn't I?'

I'm now officially famous!

After lunch, surgery started again at 2.00 and went through until 6.00, but it wasn't fully booked, so it was a bit less hectic. It was just me and Brian because Darren only worked in the morning. Brian seems like a nice enough bloke, if a little odd. He's the only vet that I've ever seen dressed in a three-piece pin-striped suit! Apparently he was at college with Darren and Paul, but only recently started working for them when they started this weekend scheme. He told me that he'd just come back from a couple of months neutering cats in Greece, which sounded quite good fun – working in the morning and sunbathing all afternoon. No chance of that in wet, grey Halesowen!

I'm on call tonight. I hope it's quiet because if tomorrow is anything like today, I'm going to need all the sleep I can get.

Sunday 9 November

4.16 a.m. I can't believe it! Some woman has just rung me up to ask for some advice about her cat, which is shaking its ears. I seriously think that people assume that the on-duty vet is up and awake all night, answering the phones. Some people are quite surprised when I answer the phone really sleepily – 'Oh, did I wake you up?' they say, obviously expecting me to be awake, alert and busily on duty.

I don't mind being woken up for a true emergency, but to be woken up and asked whether it's normal for a cat to be shaking and rubbing its ears is bloody annoying. Especially when I know full well that the cat has probably been shaking its ears for days, but the owner has only got around to ringing when it's convenient to her.

9.05 a.m. Damn! I got dressed, had some breakfast, all ready to start consulting, and then I remembered that Darren said surgery doesn't start until 10.00 on Sundays. Back to bed for half an hour. I might even get a bit of peace because the cleaners have gone.

9.15 a.m. Got an emergency coming down! A woman just rang up and said her husband has just run over their dog, so I told her to bring it straight up to the surgery.

9.50 a.m. Bit of an anticlimax really. I was expecting broken bones, collapsed lungs, bleeding lacerations, etc., but instead a bruised foot was the extent of the injuries. I felt pleased for the dog (nice two-year-old springer spaniel called Jess) but at the same time slightly disappointed that I wasn't going to get to do some exciting surgery or valiantly save the dog with emergency medicine. I always feel guilty when I get disappointed by a case like this, which sounds as though it's going to be really interesting but actually turns out to be pretty routine. I should be pleased for the animal, not selfishly annoyed that I'm not going to get to mend a broken leg or something.

Morning surgery looks bad. I'm on my own because Brian is doing the branch surgery this morning, and there are about fifteen people booked in between now and 12.00.

1.10 p.m. That was bad! Not only was I over-fully booked anyway, but about three extras turned up without appointments. When I'm busy like that, I get so irrationally annoyed by people just coming in and expecting to be seen. I shouldn't get so worked up really, because that's what the surgery is there for, and if the animal needs to be seen, then it needs to be seen. Some people do come in with trivial problems ('Oh, little Mitzi's claws need clipping, I just can't bear to see her like this any more, the poor little angel') and expect to be seen straight away, which does get me angry. I always end up seeing them, though, and however hard I try to be fierce and tell them off for not having an appointment, I can never do it and end up being much too friendly!

People can get very funny about not being seen when they want to. In Leicester, I answered the phone to a woman who demanded an appointment that morning at exactly 10.00. When I said that we were actually fully booked and the earliest available appointment was 11.20, she got really upset and started ranting on about how important it was that her dog was seen earlier, and that she had an appointment at the hairdresser's at 11.00, so that was no good. In the end she said she'd have to leave it and that she'd be complaining to Barry when he returned (a sure sign of an awkward client is one who calls the boss by his first name). I just can't believe people are so unreasonable – she should try and get a doctor's appointment at such short notice and see what happens.

Afternoon surgery isn't looking so terrible at the moment, but I'm sure it'll fill up in the next hour. I'm off to try and find some lunch.

6.10 p.m. Good afternoon. Not too busy, and a few interesting cases. The best was a big chocolate Labrador which had been playing with a stick and had managed to skewer himself on it. The stick had gone into the side of his mouth (from the inside), and when I examined him, all I could see was a large hole with some splinters of wood poking out.

I anaesthetized him once the surgery rush had calmed down (Brian was back by this point as well), and spent about twenty minutes picking bits of wood out of the wound and exploring it to make sure there weren't any splinters tracking deeper in. One of the risks with injuries like this is that bits of wood can get forced deep into the neck and damage all the big nerves and blood vessels, which run quite close to the back of the mouth. If a bit of wood was left in and the wound closed, it could migrate around in the neck, leaving a trail of infection and damage, which could end up being life-threatening.

I was pretty confident that I managed to get all the wood out, and then after flushing the wound out, I sutured it closed. He went home just now, looking good. As long as I didn't miss any bits of wood, he should be fine. His owners should have learnt the lesson that it's not a good idea to throw sticks for dogs.

Now I've just got the hour and a half drive back to Bristol!

Tuesday 11 November

We've just heard that we can move into a bungalow in Cheltenham this weekend.

Emma's had to commute from Tim's to her new job for the last week, which has been really tiring for her. The job is great, though, she's really enjoying it. I think she's just happy to be working somewhere where small-animal work isn't considered an annoying interruption to the large-animal work. Because it was a traditional large-animal practice in Dulverton, the small-animal work was quite limited and the facilities relatively basic. Although she enjoyed a lot of the large-animal work, her real interest is definitely in small animals, especially surgery. Her new practice is 100 per cent small-animal and has excellent facilities, so hopefully she'll be much happier and get to do more of the kind of work she really enjoys. Already, in her first week, she said she's done far more surgery than she used to do in a week in Dulverton, and although she's having to work pretty hard, she's finding it rewarding. Meanwhile, I'm spending the week sorting out all our stuff and trying out some new ideas on the grassboard. I've found a company in Bristol who can make the rubber bushes which I need, so it's all starting to come together.

The other thing I found while I was sorting out all our

stuff was the book I was writing. I read through it and have decided that it was in fact pretty crap and not really worth carrying on with. However, my literary career may not be over yet, because I've had another idea for a novel – a comedy about a hapless vet, who blunders his way through work and life in general, and then one day gets caught up in some serious plot. I'm not quite sure what kind of serious plot, but I'll work on that bit.

Friday 14 November

Went surfing yesterday, for the first time in ages. The surf was excellent – about five foot and lovely and clean with a gentle off-shore breeze – and because it was a Thursday there were only about five other people out, which is almost unheard of for Croyde on such a good day.

I got back to find a message on Tim's answerphone from Mrs MacNauton at Manor Vets. She wanted to know if I could work next weekend (the 22nd and 23rd), and possibly do a few weekdays as well, because they're a bit short staffed at the moment.

I rang her back and confirmed the weekend and also the one afterwards and a couple of days in the week. I need all the work I can get because Emma doesn't get paid until the end of the month and we're completely out of money.

Still no jobs in the *Vet Record* near Cheltenham.

Saturday 15 November

8.00 a.m. We've got a hectic day of moving in front of us. Well, to be more precise, *I've* got a hectic day of moving in front of *me*! Emma's managed to ensure that she's working this morning, so she said there was no point in her coming back to Bristol just to help me load the van!

The BBC are coming to film the move (the next series has definitely been commissioned because the one that's going out at the moment is doing really well). I can't quite see why people would want to see us move, but Amanda assured me it would make scintillating TV, so who am I to argue?

11.20 a.m. One hired van packed full. The last thing in was my old foam mattress, which I rescued from a skip about three years ago and have been holding on to ever since. I've got this vain hope that one day I'll get a van that I can convert into a surf-wagon for weekends and holidays, and I'll need the mattress for the bed! It'll probably never happen, but I just can't bring myself to throw it away. Emma hates it with a passion, and keeps trying to get rid of it surreptitiously whenever we move our stuff. It's come this far, though, so I'm not giving up on it now – I will have my surf-wagon. Oh, yes!

The camera crew filmed the loading, and even helped in between takes. They nearly got a good animal story as well, because there was a cat loitering around while I was loading the van, and I very nearly drove off with it curled up on my beloved mattress! Luckily it couldn't take the damp odour of the foam for very long and decided to get out before it was overcome by the fumes!

4.00 p.m. The bungalow, Cheltenham We're in! It feels great finally to have our own place together and not be either forty miles apart, or crammed into a tiny room with all our stuff. The bungalow is OK, but the decoration is pretty ghastly – the walls are covered in floral wallpaper, which is not quite to our taste, to say the least. It's much better than anywhere we've lived before, though, so I think we can put up with a bit of dodgy decoration.

It's in a good location, tucked away behind a hotel in a little mini-cul-de-sac, and is only about five minutes' walk from Emma's practice and shops and pubs (obviously the most important thing). The dog walking is the only real problem. There is a good playing field about five minutes away, but otherwise we'll have to drive out into the country to give them a good run. The dogs seem to approve of our new house; they both ran straight up to the door and waited expectantly for us to let them in and then, when we let them into the garden, they marked out their new territory with little squirts of wee, as if to say, 'Yup, this is OK. We'll take it.'

Amanda has just produced a bottle of champagne for us as a moving-in present, which we thought was a lovely gesture – until she said that she wanted to film us drinking it in our new house. They're a cunning lot, the BBC, oiling the wheels of this so-called 'fly on the wall' documentary with bottles of bubbly – not that we're complaining!

Sunday 16 November

11.15 a.m. Lovely lie in. The old mattress saved the day, because we realized yesterday that we didn't have a bed. Emma threatened to sleep on the floor rather than on the mattress, but in the end she gave in and even had to agree in the morning that it was very comfortable (if a little musty).

The dogs are demanding their breakfasts so I'm going to have to get up – Emma's claimed bed privilege because she's been working all week.

4.30 p.m. Great, relaxing day. It's so good being together in our own space. Much as I like Tim and Nicky, it was getting a bit cramped in their flat.

We've just got back from walking the mutts up on a fantastic place called Cleeve Hill, which is just north of Cheltenham. Not only is it a great dog-walking place, but it looks like grassboarding heaven! It's got beautiful smooth slopes, with steep bits and perfect-looking jumps and drop-offs; I can't wait to have a go on it. I'm not sure whether I'll be allowed or not, but I'll have a go and see if I get thrown off. There's a big sign at the bottom of the hill that states what is and isn't permitted, and grassboarding isn't mentioned! I just hope that it doesn't count as a 'Cart or carriage' because the use of them on the hill is expressly forbidden, as is 'Biking' and 'Motorized Vehicles of all types'.

Thursday 20 November

2.30 p.m. I've spent the last few days sorting out the house, apart from a big pile of boxes in the front room which I can't face unpacking, and experimenting with the grassboard.

I had a big grassboard crisis on Tuesday, because I tried it out at Cleeve Hill and it wasn't working at all well. The problem was that because Cleeve Hill is a bit steeper than most of the other places I've tried it on, its lack of tight turning ability was really exposed and meant I couldn't turn quickly enough to stay in control. There are a couple of great-looking runs which should be fantastic, with banks on either side to jump off, which I just couldn't get down because the board couldn't turn tightly enough. I ended up getting really depressed about it, thinking that after all my effort and expectations, the idea was doomed to failure.

I spent that evening working out ways in which I could increase the turning ability of the board without moving away from the principle of how it works (the flex and lean of the board creating the turn) and ending up like the MBS rival. Eventually, after toying with various ideas, I worked out that the simplest way to improve it would be to angle the ends of the board up. This, I figured, should effectively act to increase the angle between the two axles when the board is tilted, thus making the turning circle much tighter.

I spent most of yesterday, and this morning, working in the garage, trying to alter the end of the board to solve the problem, and I think I've finally got it sorted. Now I'm off to Cleeve Hill for a test run.

4.40 p.m. Grassboard is back on track! The alterations made all the difference. Now I can manoeuvre it much better, and I made it down all the runs I couldn't get down on Tuesday. I'm going to be a millionaire after all!

10.30 p.m. Early night because my life of luxury is over – I'm working at Manor tomorrow and the weekend.

Friday 21 November

7.00 a.m. Urrumph!

7.40 a.m. Leaving house. I'm not used to being up at this time of the morning, let alone having to face over an hour's drive and a full day's work.

8.35 a.m. Manor Vet Centre, Halesowen The traffic on the M5 was a nightmare. Emma's car kept almost overheating, so I spent the entire journey alternating between worrying about being late for work and worrying whether the car would make it or not. Emma blew the engine up while she was working in Dulverton, and ever since the rebuild it's not been quite right. We need to sell it and get a cheaper, but more reliable, car. We should be so lucky!

9.00 a.m. When I arrived, I went up to the vets' room and had a cup of coffee with Paul and Darren. They discussed a few of the ongoing cases, and updated me on some of the ones I'd seen the previous weekend. The dog with the stick injury was fine, so that means I must have managed to get all the bits out OK, but there's one case I saw which has deteriorated over the last week. It's another Labrador, called Max, and when I saw him he was just a little off-colour and lethargic. Darren said that since then he'd gradually got worse, and was now really weak and poorly. He's booked in this morning, so I'll see how he's getting on.

1.30 p.m. Hectic morning surgery again. I think I saw about twenty people, which is pretty hard going for a three-and-a-half-hour surgery.

Max the poorly Labrador came in, and he's really declined. He's only about nine years old, but he looks ancient. He's gone thin and his coat is really dull. His owners are a nice young couple called Mr and Mrs Hanks, and they're understandably concerned.

'He's just not himself at all,' said Mr Hanks, in the Brummie accent I'm becoming accustomed to. 'This morning we offered him some ham and he just sniffed at it and walked away, didn't he, love?'

'Mm,' agreed his wife, obviously close to tears. 'He normally loves his ham, don't you, Max?'

She reached down to pat him and, as she did so, the flood-gates opened and she burst into tears.

'Oh, I'm so sorry,' she sobbed, 'you must think I'm stupid, getting all upset like this, but he's such a good boy, and I couldn't stand it if we lost him.'

I tried to comfort her as best I could, and said that we'd keep him in for the moment to try and find out what was going on. It really moved me, seeing how upset she was, Max obviously means so much to her.

3.30 p.m. I've got Max on a drip, and taken some blood. They haven't got a blood machine here, so it'll have to go off to the lab, but we should still get a result tomorrow morning. I asked Darren why such a good practice hadn't got a blood analyser, and he said that he felt that the results from the machines weren't always as accurate as when the tests are done in a lab. I suppose he's probably right, but it's still a little frustrating to have to wait twenty-four hours for the results, however accurate they are.

I told him that I have a suspicion as to Max's problem. I think he might have a tumour in his abdomen which is bleeding, causing him to be weak and pale. It fits in with his symptoms: the gradual deterioration, the lethargy and general malaise. I hope I'm wrong, because if that is the case, it may well be inoperable. There is a chance that if there is a tumour inside, we might be able to remove it, but quite often they spread and there's little that can be done.

Darren agreed it was a possibility, but said there wasn't really enough evidence to consider doing an exploratory operation yet, and it would be better to wait for the blood results before rushing into anything. I know he's right, and my theory is really little more than a hunch, but I hope that by delaying, we don't miss a chance to save him. It's a hard decision to make, because if we do operate, there is a chance he won't survive the anaesthetic in his weakened state, and if I'm wrong and there is no tumour, I'll have put him through the risky operation for nothing. On the other hand, if we leave him and my suspicions are correct, he could die before we get round to opening him up. I think I'll listen to Darren's advice because he's much more experienced than I am – I tend to get an idea and convince myself it's right, whereas I should sit back and look at the evidence more objectively and take my time more.

I've told the Hankses that we'll keep him in overnight and see how he is tomorrow, when we should get the blood results back. At least here, although it's not officially a hospital practice, they have a nurse on duty all the time who comes in to check on the animals at night and is on duty for emergencies, so I feel confident that he'll be looked after through the night.

Evening surgery starts at 4.30, so I'm off to grab a belated lunch before getting on with another three-hour consulting marathon.

7.30 p.m. Finally finished! It's been a very hard work day, but I've really enjoyed it. I've seen lots of interesting cases, and I've also learnt quite a lot from talking things over with Darren and Paul. They're both really involved in their work, and it's good to work somewhere like this, where everyone works well as a team and gets on with each other. This is the first practice I've been to where there are no obvious undercurrents of discontent between the staff. All the nurses are nice and don't spend all day bitching about each other, which is very unusual!

I really feel as though my enthusiasm for being a vet is being reawakened again, after getting a bit disillusioned over the last six months. Working here is the perfect antidote for the time I spent in Leicester. After that week I thought being a vet was maybe not for me, and seeing the state of the practice almost killed off any enthusiasm for the job I had. Now I feel as though I've rediscovered what being a vet is all about – working in a happy, well-organized, high-quality practice has made me realize that being a vet can be fun and interesting and it's what I want to keep doing.

Sunday 23 November

9.15 a.m. Yesterday was hectic, but ended up being very rewarding. We got the blood results back from Max at about 11.00. There were no obvious abnormalities except for the fact that his red blood cell count was really low. This was the first piece of solid evidence to support my bleeding abdominal tumour theory, so I was keen to look for any more clues which might confirm the diagnosis and allow me to get on and operate.

After morning surgery had finished I took a couple of X-rays of his abdomen which were fairly inconclusive. There was no sign of any large masses, but I was not really expecting any such clear-cut findings, because I'd had a good feel of his abdomen and couldn't palpate anything. There was, however, some loss of contrast and blurring of the detail throughout the ventral abdomen, and I knew this could be consistent with blood or other fluid loss. But I still didn't have enough evidence to warrant an exploratory operation, especially as Max was very weak, and his low red blood cell count would make any operation much more risky.

I spent a few minutes watching him, lying quietly in his kennel, with a drip in his leg. He occasionally lifted his head and looked up with a mournful expression which seemed to be saying, 'Well, come on then, find out what's wrong with me, I haven't got all day you know!'

I was beginning to realize he really didn't have all day. He was starting to look weaker and weaker, and his colour was now a dangerously pale shade of pink.

I sat there looking at him and tried to think rationally about the facts of the case, and wondered whether or not I should take the plunge and act on my impulse diagnosis without any real firm proof. Then I realized there was one more diagnostic test I could try in order to confirm my theory. I ran out of the kennels and found Emma, one of the nurses, and between us we carried Max out to the examination table in the prep room. I clipped and sterilized a small area of skin about four inches behind his ribs, in the midline, and then placed a small blob of local anaesthetic under the skin.

'What are you going to do, Joe?' Emma asked, as I rummaged through the needle drawer looking for a long narrow hypodermic needle.

'I'm going to try abdominocentesis to see if there is any blood in the abdomen. If we do get some blood back then I think I must be right about him having a bleeding tumour inside.'

'Oh. Right,' she replied, obviously unconvinced.

As I slipped the inch-and-a-half-long needle through the anaesthetized muscles of Max's abdominal wall, I hoped I was right, and that when I pulled back on the syringe, blood would come back. I felt I needed to prove myself to some degree both to the nurses and to Darren and the other vets. It's all very well trying to get on with everyone as much as possible, but unless they respect you as a competent vet then you're never going to really fit in at a practice. I felt this here especially because of the overall quality of the staff. I really didn't want to be wrong on such an important diagnosis so soon after starting work.

I pulled back on the syringe and looked in dismay as nothing was drawn up. I repositioned the needle slightly and tried again and to my immense relief the barrel of the syringe suddenly filled up with pale-looking blood.

I withdrew the needle and turned triumphantly to Emma and Darren who'd just come in.

'Look's like you were right,' said Darren. 'Are you going to open him up then?'

'Yes, I don't think we've got a choice really, have we? Will I be all right to do that this afternoon, if there's only me and Brian on?' I asked, thinking about how I could fit the op in as well as consult all afternoon.

'Just wait until you've done the busy hour or so after lunch and then crack on with it,' he advised. 'Let's just keep our fingers crossed that it's something you can remove.'

By this time afternoon surgery was just starting, so I grabbed a quick sandwich and got on with the consulting. At about 3.15, the worst of the surgery was over, so I checked that Brian was OK to carry on on his own ('Yes, no worries, you get on with it'), and started to get things ready for the op.

Emma, like all the nurses here, was helpful and encouraging as I prepared the anaesthetic and the instruments. It's so nice to have nurses who know what they're doing and who make operating so much easier and less stressful. The difference between working with the nurses here and the nurses in Leicester is like taking your car to a modern, professional garage, where everything is done quickly and to a high standard, and having an MOT at a dodgy back-street garage where they weld stolen cars together as a sideline!

I used a short-acting anaesthetic injection, so that Max would wake up as quickly as possible after the operation and then, once he was asleep, Emma held his head up so I could slide the endo-tracheal tube into his windpipe. Emma connected the tube to the anaesthetic circuit and stabilized him on the gas, which would keep him asleep through the operation.

After I scrubbed up, Emma handed me a sterile packet containing a long-sleeved gown and a separate packet containing sterile operating gloves. I hadn't used a sterile gown and gloves since leaving college, apart from the odd occasion in Bideford, so it took me a while to struggle my way into them without contaminating the gown or my hands. Putting on sterile gloves using the correct method is the real test of any vet. You are supposed carefully to hook part of the glove over the thumb of the first hand before putting on the second glove with a special manoeuvre which involves all sorts of strange hand contortions. The idea is to minimize any contamination of the gloves by less than sterile hands, but I have yet to master it with any degree of success. I end up getting both gloves stuck half on and have to spend the next twenty minutes gradually easing the fingers on, only to get to the last finger which tears as I try to ease it over a fingernail! At vet school I think the average student used to get through about three or four pairs of gloves per operation, and I've yet to meet a vet to this day who claims to be able to master the correct gloving-up technique.

Anyway, I was eventually ready, sterile from head to toe, and Emma pronounced Max safely anaesthetized, so I started the operation. The nerves which I'd felt when drawing the blood from his abdomen returned with a vengeance as I cut through his dark skin and the muscles below – what if I was wrong after all and there was no tumour? What if I'd waited too long and he died before we finished the op?

I opened up the abdomen and immediately a rush of bloody fluid spilt out of it and started pouring on to the drapes surrounding the wound. Emma quickly placed a bowl on the floor to collect the fluid as it dripped off the edge of the table, but I was too slow to stop a large red stain appearing on the front of my gown.

It took a few minutes to clear most of the pint or two of fluid which had accumulated in the abdomen, but once the field was clear I was able to examine the abdominal organs in the search for the source of this bleeding.

My first stop was the spleen, because this is by far the most common site for bleeding abdominal tumours in older dogs, but when I pulled the smooth, flat, blueish coloured organ from the abdomen I could find no sign of the irregular, haemorrhagic mass that I was expecting. Next I examined the thin tissue-like mesentery, which carries the blood vessels to the intestines, but again there was no sign of any tumours or other causes of bleeding.

I finally found what I was looking for on the liver. As I ran my fingers over its smooth surface, I felt a small, soft mass attached to one lobe, deep in the abdomen. As I brought the mass to the surface to examine it more closely, I felt relief and excitement take over from nervous expectation. If this small mass was the only source of the bleeding, and if the rest of the liver was OK, then there was a chance that I could remove it and Max would pull through.

I gently eased the edge of the liver up to the light and saw the dark mass that I'd felt attached to the tip of the rounded, tan-coloured liver lobe. The mass was about an inch in diameter and was obviously the source of some, if not all, of the bleeding, because its irregular surface was covered in a mixture of fresh and clotted blood. As I touched the mass, I could see new bleeding starting as the friable tissue disintegrated beneath my fingers.

I'd never attempted any sort of liver surgery before, so this was new territory for me. I remembered my lecture notes saying that because the liver is so delicate, it's very hard to suture, so in most cases all that can be done is to crush and tear the tissue.

'Would you like some Calcistat?' asked Emma, opening

the glass cupboard which contained the suture materials and drugs.

'Er, can you just remind me exactly what that is?' I'd never heard of Calcistat, but it sounded very useful.

'It stops bleeding,' Emma explained, opening a small packet and handing me a piece of white material which looked like soft white cardboard.

'Ah, yes. I know,' I lied, figuring that I could work out how it was used and save some face at least.

Armed with the Calcistat, I gently worked the mass free of the liver. Once it was off, I pressed a piece of the white material over the oozing edge of the liver and hoped that this was what you were supposed to do with it. I looked confidently at Emma, half expecting her to shout out, 'No, no! What are you doing? You can't just put it on like that!' and call Darren through to sort out the mess I'd made, but it looked like I'd guessed right. When I turned back to the wound, I could see the bleeding had all but stopped; so after checking the rest of the liver over carefully for other masses, I let it slip gently back into the abdomen.

I waited a while to check that no blood was filling the abdomen up again, and once I was happy, I sutured the wound up. All in all, the operation had taken just over an hour.

I sent the mass off to the lab for analysis so we can give the Hankses some idea of whether it's likely to recur or spread. There was no sign of any secondary tumours in the abdomen, so hopefully the results will show that it was a benign tumour and that will be that – problem solved.

I'm so happy that my diagnosis was right and that the op went well. If he survives, it'll be one of the best cases I've had.

6.00 p.m. Busy all day again today, lots of routine cases with the occasional interesting ones, such as a budgie with pink swellings in its eyes and a cat with an airgun pellet under its skin. Max has improved throughout the day and is now sitting up in his kennel, wagging his tail. I've told Mr and Mrs Hanks that he should be OK to go home tomorrow as long as there are no complications. They were so happy when I explained how everything had gone – they said they really hadn't expected to see him alive again after they left him yesterday morning.

Home to Cheltenham now, thank God. It's been an excellent weekend, but bloody knackering to say the least.

Monday 24 November

10.00 a.m. Just rang up Halesowen to see how Max is this morning, and they said he was fine, and Mrs Hanks is coming in to pick him up this afternoon.

I'm going to spend the day sorting out the garage. I think I'd almost rather be at work!

3.15 p.m. Amanda from the BBC has just rung and asked if they can come and film this weekend in Halesowen. I told her they should have been there last weekend, because Max would have been a good story for them to follow. I suppose I see so many more cases each day there than I ever did in Devon that they shouldn't have any problem finding enough things to film.

I mentioned the BBC filming to Darren last weekend and he was really keen. I think that he can see the commercial benefits of the free advertising!

Wednesday 26 November

Exciting news left, right and centre!!

The press officer from the BBC rang up this morning and asked if Emma would like to be on *Richard and Judy* next week! Apparently there's loads of interest in the series, and loads of newspapers and shows want interviews and photos of people. Neither of us can believe we're actually going to appear on live morning TV!

And, as if that wasn't enough, he also said that the *Daily Express* wants to do a feature on us as a couple, and gave us the number of one of the journalists! I rang her up today and she was really nice, and explained exactly what she wanted to write (it sounds quite cheesy, but who cares? It'll be amazing enough to have a feature on us in a national paper). She's going to do the interview over the phone tonight.

6.30 p.m. Just finished my part of the interview and handed the phone over to Emma. It was OK, mainly questions like, 'How long have you wanted to be a vet?' and, 'How did you and Emma meet?' No investigative probing into unexplained pheasant deaths in North Devon or sudden hamster deaths, which was a relief!

6.45 p.m. Emma's done. I didn't listen to most of her answers, but when I came back into the room at the end, I did hear her saying ' . . . bit of a disappointment really.' She claimed that she was talking about the Langford job that she didn't get, but I'm not sure I believe her!

Friday 28 November

A woman from the *Richard and Judy* office has just rung up and confirmed all the details for our appearance next Wednesday. We're not getting a fee, but they're paying for all our expenses, including staying overnight in a hotel in London. It should be great fun.

Saturday 29 November

1.30 p.m. I arrived late this morning thanks to a five-mile tailback on the M5. When I finally made it, at about 9.00, the waiting room was packed with owners, animals, and the

BBC crew. Amanda, Emma and new camera- and soundmen (Rob and Paul) were waiting for me, but there was no time for lengthy introductions or for me to show them around, because the waiting list on my computer screen already had four people on it.

I didn't leave the consulting room, except for a quick wee break at about 11.00, until the last client was seen at about 12.30. Every time I finished one consultation, two or three new clients appeared on the waiting list, so I just had to plough on. Even for this place it seemed exceptionally busy – usually there's at least a few five-minute gaps between patients through the morning. I found out why it was so busy when I finally got out of the consulting room and saw who was working with me – Mrs MacNauton was one of the other vets on this morning, but as far as I could gather, she'd not come down from her office at all. I suppose that's the advantage of being the boss, but it seems a bit unfair of her to sit upstairs doing office work or whatever she does while her minions slave away below.

The other vet on for the weekend is a bloke called Martin who I'd not met before. As soon as I saw him come out of his consulting room I thought, Oh, no! It's Neil Tomkins back to haunt me! But then I realized that although he does look quite similar to the infamous first-year anatomy lecturer, he doesn't have that same superior, eyes-half-closed patronizing manner which characterized Neil. In general appearance they are quite similar though, both mid-thirties with short, messy, light-brown hair and pale skin. He seems like a nice enough bloke, if a little reserved. I did get out of him the fact that he'd just moved from a referral centre in Leeds where he did high-powered orthopaedic surgery, and that he's not quite sure what he's planning to do next, so he's doing these weekends to make ends meet for a while.

The BBC filmed a few cases, but it was really too busy for them to get any decent stories. Maybe this afternoon will be a bit quieter and we'll have some decent cases in for them to follow.

3.00 p.m. The lab have just faxed through the result of Max Hanks' lump analysis. It turns out it was a nasty tumour called a haemangiosarcoma, and according to the pathologist at the lab, it could well have already spread and may come back. I phoned Mr Hanks and explained what the results meant, and he seemed to take it fairly well. He said that Max is doing great at the moment and if there's any sign of his symptoms returning they'll bring him straight down. I hope it doesn't return, but I have a nasty feeling Max's days may be numbered. Tumours like this are usually pretty aggressive and I won't be surprised if another one starts causing problems pretty soon. You never know, though, maybe he'll live on happily for years to come.

At least he's better now and, even if he doesn't last too much longer, we've given him a few extra weeks or months of decent life.

7.30 p.m. The BBC are taking me out for a meal. I'm on call and I've got my phone with me so I can always rush back if there's an emergency.

This afternoon was better, not so busy, and we had a couple of good cases in. The best one was a woman who brought in an English bull terrier pup which she'd found abandoned by the roadside. It was about six months old and in a terrible state. Instead of a nice white coat, the pup was covered in horrible red scabs and lesions all over her face, ears, legs and belly.

I checked her over and, apart from her skin problems, she was a little thin but otherwise in reasonable health. The woman who had found her, Mrs Ball, had decided that if she was OK, she would take her on and give her a home.

'I just can't believe that anyone could just leave her there, on the side of a main road,' she said, stroking the puppy, who was sitting quietly on the consulting table.

'I wouldn't stroke her too much,' I warned her. 'I think she's probably got mange, and it might be one that can be passed to humans. What I'll do is take a few skin scrapings and have a look under the microscope, and then I'll be able to say if it is mange or not, and if it is, which type.'

I took the scrapings with a scalpel blade and some liquid paraffin, and placed the slide under the microscope. I've done this lots of times since I qualified, but very rarely have I actually seen any mites, so I was expecting to have to hunt around for a while to find anything. However, as soon as I focused the microscope on the slide, I could see three elongated cigar-shaped creatures with tiny legs filling the field of view – Demodex mites without a doubt.

I went back to the consulting room to tell Mrs Ball the diagnosis. It was good to be able to say exactly what the problem was, without any further tests, and say that we should be able to cure the dog completely. I told her in detail about the mites and how we could treat them with anti-mite washes. I also said that this type of mange isn't contagious to humans, and rarely spreads between animals. It's mainly spread from mother to offspring.

I sent her away with a bottle of potent anti-mite wash, anti-bacterial shampoo and antibiotic tablets to clear up the secondary skin infection, and asked her to come back every week for a month or so for check-ups to make sure it clears up OK.

I remember reading a James Herriot story where he's faced with a group of dogs with mange and he can't do anything for them. It must have been so frustrating in those days to be faced with diseases like that and have no effective treatments, and to have to watch the animals suffer until, in some cases, they died from the disease. Modern vets tend to take a lot of treatments for granted and forget how easily treatable diseases today were incurable killers just a few years ago. It's amazing reading about life as a vet in the thirties and forties because, in most ways, it's so far removed from modern practice. But there are still a lot of things which never change, like clients who ring up in the middle of the night for trivial problems, and the animals themselves. Modern medicine and surgery may be almost unrecognizable from how it was fifty years ago, but modern cats and dogs are just the same as they've always been.

Sunday 30 November

9.30 a.m. Quiet night, busy day ahead.

8.30 p.m. Cheltenham Home sweet home! Very happy to be back. Although I'm still really enjoying working in Halesowen, the one thing I hate is having to stay up there in the flat on Saturday night to be on call.

Mrs MacNauton came in this afternoon and asked me if I could start doing some weekdays because one of their full-time vets has just left and they're short-staffed. I said that I'd love to – we need all the money we can get. Also it'll be good to do some operating because I'm just consulting most of the time at the weekends, except for the occasional emergency like Max Hanks.

I'm doing tomorrow and Thursday. She wanted me to work Wednesday as well but I explained that we were off to London for *Richard and Judy*!

December

Tuesday 2 December

Good day at Halesowen yesterday. I operated in the morning, which made a change from consulting all the time. It was still really hard work, though, I was used to doing three or four ops in a morning at Bideford, but I did nine yesterday morning.

bitch spay (nice easy border collie)
two cat spays
one dog castration
one cystotomy (only the second one I've ever done; removed a massive jagged stone from the bladder of a poor old sheltie, very satisfying)
two dentals (one horrible cat, one horrible Yorkie; the Yorkie started the op with a mouth full of rotten teeth and ended up with only one tooth left)
stitch up cat's paw (ripped on glass, neat wound, stitched up nicely)
lump removal (very small wart under eye on poodle, owners more worried by the dog's looks than its health)

We're off to London this afternoon. A taxi is coming to pick us up and take us to the station, and another one should meet us in London and take us to our hotel. I could certainly get used to the life of a celebrity.

Wednesday 3 December

9.15 p.m. What an experience! It's been an excellent twenty-four hours to say the least!

We got to London at about 7 p.m. last night, and were taken to the Marriot Hotel. We couldn't believe it when the taxi stopped outside the front doors of this enormous, posh-looking mansion – we were expecting to be put up in a little

313

cheap hotel or Travelodge on some motorway service station, not to be taken to a massive, glittering hotel in St John's Wood.

Our room was by far the best hotel room that either of us has ever stayed in – we've been more used to finding the cheapest B&B or seediest hotel whenever we've had to stay somewhere because of our meagre student budgets, so finding that we had a bed the size of a small football field, a TV with satellite channels, and a glorious power-shower was so exciting!

After trying the bedroom out thoroughly (the TV and shower, I mean), we wandered down to the dining room. We immediately felt completely out of place: there we were dressed in our scruffy jeans and T-shirts, while everyone else was smartly attired in suits and posh dresses. We were shown to the most distant table in the room by a haughty waiter and presented with a menu. We decided that since ITV were paying, we really ought to have the most expensive food and wine available, so we ordered a fantastic meal of succulent beef medallions, Atlantic prawns and a bottle of the most expensive wine on the menu. The food was good but unfortunately the wine was grim. Neither of us was confident enough to complain, though, because we weren't entirely sure whether the wine was supposed to taste like a bottle of malt vinegar to which someone had added some warm urine or not. We battled through it and moved on to safer ground with a few pints of Stella.

This morning we were again picked up by a taxi and driven to Television Studios on the South Bank, where we were met by the woman who we'd spoken to on the phone, Nadia. She, like everyone else we saw all morning, was rushing around, continually talking into a headset and generally giving off an air of low-level panic.

We were shown into the Green Room, which is the room where the guests are supposed to relax before going on the show. It wasn't green at all, and we certainly *didn't* relax. I was getting more and more nervous as we waited and watched the show on a monitor. About half an hour before we were due on, we were taken through into make-up and both of us were covered in foundation and various other colours and creams. When I came out I felt like someone had poured some wet concrete on my face – I don't know how women can wear thick layers of make-up every day. Emma was just as unused to wearing an inch of Max Factor's best because her idea of getting made-up is to apply a tiny bit of mascara (which I think is much better than wearing loads of make-up – women should be happy with their features as they are, not plaster themselves in make-up).

Then, all of a sudden, we were whisked through into the studio and sat down in a mocked-up vet surgery which had been specially made on the set, complete with a basket full of kittens mewing in the corner. Richard and Judy came over and said hello and seemed very nice and friendly, and then, before we could ask any questions, the lights dimmed and people started counting down and shouting things like, 'Thirty seconds to air' and, 'Get those cats back, now!'

Before we were on, the show started with a mad woman who thought she could talk in cat! She read the titles of the show in fluent cat – 'Meow, meoow, purr, purrrr, meow' etc., with subtitles in English below. She was completely barking mad (or should that be meowing mad!), sitting on the couch dressed in a pink dressing gown, making unrealistic cat noises. I suppose I'm being a little harsh on her because one of the kittens in the basket next to me did sit up and whisper, 'She's not bad, but I wish she'd get rid of that awful Siamese accent.'

Anyway, once the mad cat woman was finished, Richard and Judy came over and introduced us. The worst part was speaking for the first time, because I knew my voice was wavering and sounded nervous, but once we got into the swing of the interview, we both started to relax a bit and, by the end, we were talking quite well and didn't look too silly (saying that, I've just watched it on video, and I had to hide behind the sofa it was so cringe-worthy!).

Then it was all over, we were thanked and ushered out to the waiting taxi, which took us off to the station and back to dull old reality.

It was a great experience though. Live TV is so much more nerve-racking than being filmed for *Vets in Practice*. I think it's because you know that if you say something stupid, or do something silly, there's no editing to save you, the nation will see it all as it happens. I also had this horrible fear that I would suddenly swear really loudly, but thankfully I didn't!

I hope we get to do some more things like this, because it's really exciting and different to everyday life as a vet. We should try and enjoy the fruits of minor fame as much as we can because it's an opportunity few people get, and it'll probably all be over in a year or so.

10.15 p.m. Nigel, the kitten, has just come through the cat-flap carrying what looks like a fox-shaped hand puppet!

10.18 p.m. On closer inspection it definitely *is* a fox-shaped hand puppet! I wonder where the little klepto-cat got that from!

Friday 5 December

3.00 p.m. Emma's just rushed in from work really upset. Her mum's just rung her and said that Penny, her old dog, has suddenly gone downhill and is in a really bad state. Emma asked her boss if she could go home, which he said was fine, so we're heading off to Kent. From the sound of things, Emma's probably going to have to put her to sleep, which is going to be awful.

10.30 p.m. Kent Not a happy evening. We arrived at about 6.00 after a miserable journey, and were greeted by Emma's parents and sisters, who were all obviously upset and tense. I wasn't used to seeing them like this, because they're normally such a happy, cheerful family, so I felt quite awkward and didn't quite know what to do with myself.

Penny was lying on the carpet when we came in, and barely lifted her head to say hello. I'm not sure if she even recognized Emma. In the past she was always so happy to see her old mistress when she returned, but today there wasn't even a glimmer of the old excitement in the opaque blue eyes. She just lay there, her black flanks, flecked with grey, rising and falling as she breathed, oblivious to the emotional tension around her.

'She collapsed this morning while Alice was here, and she's just been lying there all day,' explained Emma's mum, Jackie. 'I think she's had enough, don't you, Rich?'

'Mm,' he agreed, obviously upset. 'She can't go on like this.'

'Fourteen is a good old age for a collie,' I said, trying to find something comforting to say, 'and she's had a lovely life.'

'She's had a great life, haven't you, Pen?' said Emma, cuddling Penny on the floor. I could see tears in her eyes as she stroked the dog, who had been Emma's companion since she was eleven.

'I remember when she could jump a six-foot wall, and now she can't even stand up,' sobbed Emma's youngest sister.

'I know, but she's old now and she can't carry on for ever,' said Jackie, trying to comfort her daughter.

Finally, after an hour or so, the decision was made that Emma would put Penny to sleep, and she managed to compose herself sufficiently to organize the injection, scissors, surgical spirit and cotton wool which are the tools of veterinary euthanasia. I had already offered to give the injection if Emma didn't feel up to it, but she said that she wanted to do this one last thing for Penny.

It was all over very quickly, thankfully. Penny didn't fight, and the needle slipped straight into the vein without any struggle. As the injection entered her bloodstream, I looked for that expression of betrayal and dismay which had haunted me in the face of the Labrador in Bideford, but all I saw was her face relax and the final glint of life gently slip away. It was as if she realized that her struggle was over and knew that what we were doing was for her own good.

After the tears and emotion cleared, a sense of relief seemed to come over everyone. Although it was so sad to see her go, it had brought an end to her suffering, and an end to the stress and worry that her suffering had been causing the family over the last few months. We toasted her with a glass of wine, and Emma and her family spent a while talking about her life and the great pleasure she'd brought to them over the fourteen years since she'd arrived as a puppy for Emma's eleventh birthday. I'd only ever seen her as an old dog, so it was good to listen to stories of how she was as a fit, lithe young collie, who'd survived being run over twice, an operation for mammary cancer and an infected womb.

Sunday 7 December

8.00 p.m. Cheltenham We got back about an hour ago, after spending the rest of the weekend with Emma's parents. After the stresses of Friday night, the rest of the weekend was more relaxed and things gradually began to return to normal. We went to the pub last night, and ended up playing pool until about 1.00 a.m. The landlord is a great bloke called Brian, who looks like a very large, intimidating bouncer from a dodgy East End night club but is, in fact, really nice and friendly (I wouldn't cross him though). He and his wife Barbara run the pub, which is just around the corner from Emma's parents' house, and over the years Emma and her three sisters have worked there. As a result, Brian and Barb are close friends of the family, and Brian especially has given out lots of help and advice to all of the sisters. Emma once described Brian as the Yoda of The Royal Oak!

We ended up talking to Brian and playing pool long after most of the regulars had gone, and I could see that it was just what Emma and the rest of the family needed to help them get over the sad events of the weekend.

8.30 p.m. Just picked up the mutts from one of Emma's nurses who'd had them over the weekend. It was great to see their slobbery, licking faces again, and when I looked at Pan and Badger, I could really understand what Emma had gone through over the last few days. It may be silly and irrational but I'm so attached to our dogs, and I'm dreading the day when we have to go through this again with these two.

Wednesday 10 December

I worked yesterday and Monday, but I'm off today, which is a relief. It's been a bit of a shock, suddenly working most of the time after the last couple of months of laziness!

I'm getting into the swing of it, and getting on with the nurses and vets quite well. I think so anyway – they probably all hate me really. Now that the whole series of *Vets in Practice* has been shown (it finished last week), I'm getting recognized quite a lot by clients. Most of them say something like, 'I'm sure I've seen you before,' or, 'Don't I know you from somewhere?' rather than immediately recognizing me from the programme. It's a good feeling, though, being slightly famous!

A woman from the local Birmingham radio station rang me at work yesterday and asked whether I'd be willing to do an interview on an afternoon programme later this week. Apparently one of the people at the station had seen me on TV and heard I was working in Halesowen. The woman also seemed interested in the grassboard, which was featured in episode six, so I should get to chat about that a bit, and you never know who might be listening – it's amazing how many heads of international snowboarding companies listen to BBC Radio West Midlands!

We fixed up the interview for 2 p.m. on Friday, because I'm working tomorrow and at the weekend.

Friday 12 December

Good day at Halesowen yesterday. I operated again and did a few interesting ones, including amputating a cat's toe which was broken and horribly infected. I also watched Darren do a cruciate ligament repair on a dog's knee. The cruciate ligament is one of the ligaments which hold the knee joint together, and rupturing it is quite a common injury in animals and people. I've never done one and I told Darren that I'm keen to learn how to do them, so he suggested I watch this one, and then the next one that comes in, he'll supervise while I do it. I hope we get another one in soon, because it's quite a challenge and I'd like to do one. Emma keeps boasting about the fact that she's done three already since she's been in her new job in Cheltenham. I think she's probably getting pretty useful with a scalpel these days, but that is what she's always been most interested in, I suppose, so I shouldn't begrudge her a little surgical superiority.

Today I did the radio interview, which went fine. I talked about the filming for *Vets in Practice* and general vet stuff for a while, and then managed to steer the conversation round to the grassboard, and explained about my idea and how the development is coming on. I hope bits of publicity like this lead somewhere, because I feel I need some assistance to get it off the ground and get a decent product into production by next summer.

Em and me are going out for a few quiet pints tonight with Rachel, the nurse from Emma's practice who looked after the mutts last weekend, and her boyfriend Kevin.

Saturday 13 December

7.15 a.m. Oh, God! It's too early!

7.20 a.m. I knew that fifth pint was a mistake, but Emma insisted. Honest!

7.55 a.m. Oh, no! I must have fallen asleep again, bugger!

8.52 a.m. Halesowen I'm not looking forward to this morning, I'm hungover, tired and insufficiently breakfasted!

I'm just glad that the BBC aren't here to film me in this state. I think my TV career would be over if the great British public saw me looking like this!

12.15 p.m. Not a bad morning, considering. A solid three-hour consulting session is enough to sort out even the worst of hangovers.

One really interesting case came in a few minutes ago, a lurcher which had been kicked in the head by a horse. It had just happened, and the owner had rushed the dog straight down to the surgery.

I opened the consulting room door and immediately ushered in a portly man of about forty carrying a blood-stained dog in his arms. Blood was streaked across the man's check shirt, and his rough working jeans also bore evidence of the dog's injury. My first impression was that the dog should be dead – her whole forehead was awash with blood, and I could see that above the left eye there was a large irregular depression where the full force of the hoof must have caught the dog squarely on the forehead.

I gave the dazed dog, who was called Zoe, a quick general checkover to make sure there were no other injuries. It looked as though she'd escaped with no other obvious problems, but the wound on her head looked bad enough.

'Did you see it happen?' I asked Mr Fuller, the owner, as I examined the injury more closely.

'No, no. Me and the wife were just out walking and she

ran off somewhere. Next thing we 'ere 'er yelp and then she comes running back wi' blood all over 'er face,' he replied.

'Well, the horse must have caught her just above the eye here.' I pointed to the obvious wound. 'It looks pretty nasty, but we'll have to take some X-rays to see what the extent of the damage is. She's got some signs of concussion – her pupils are different sizes and she's a bit uncoordinated, but that should improve over the next few hours. We'll take her in now and do the X-rays and let you know what we find. I think it'd probably be best to keep her overnight, but we'll see how she goes this afternoon.'

I'm just about to X-ray her to see what damage has been done inside the skull. I can't believe that she's as well as she is considering the size of the hole in her head!

1.10 p.m. Good news. The X-ray shows that Zoe has been incredibly lucky – the kick crushed the bones over one of the big air-filled sinuses at the front of the skull which absorbed the impact, and the cranium below looks intact. A few inches higher or lower and it would have been a different story but, as it is, if the concussion resolves and we can sort out the wound, she should be OK.

I'm not quite sure what to do about the smashed skull pieces. I've cleaned up the worst of the mess and it doesn't actually look too bad. There's only one cut, which should heal on its own, and apart from that most of the damage is restricted to the shattered bits of bone underneath.

I rang Mr Fuller and said we'd keep her in tonight and make a decision on whether to try and fix the bones, remove the pieces, or just leave it as it is and let it heal, once she'd fully got over the concussion in a few days' time. In the meantime I've put her on painkillers and antibiotics, mainly as a precaution in case any infection gets in. It could turn from a lucky escape into an unlucky disaster if infection were to take hold inside the sinus, where it could spread deep into the sensitive areas below.

7.20 p.m. Sad case this afternoon. I got the blood results back from a lovely eleven-year-old collie that I'd seen on Thursday because it had some hair loss and was a bit off colour. I was expecting to find that it was hypothyroid or had some liver or kidney problems, but I wasn't expecting the diagnosis that came back. According to the haematology, the dog has leukaemia.

Before I broke the bad news to the owners I spent a while reading up on the condition because I'd never come across a case like this before. From what I remembered from university, leukaemia is a nasty, rapidly lethal disease, and animals suffering from it should be very ill. This dog is bright, alert, and just a little unwilling to run too far (which could easily just be arthritis), so to find out that it was suffering from such a nasty cancer was a very unpleasant shock.

However, according to the textbooks, it's not that uncommon to diagnose the condition with a routine blood test for something completely unrelated, because the disease can progress slowly for months or even years before any clinical symptoms become apparent. I assumed that the outlook for the dog would be pretty poor, perhaps a few months at best if we got it on chemotherapy, but again I was surprised to read that if the animal is well in itself, there is no real need to start treatment immediately and the outlook can be measured in years rather than months.

I told Mr and Mrs Hewlett when they brought Tara back in for a check this afternoon, and they seemed to take the news fairly well. I explained that although the disease could be behind the hair problems and lethargy, unless she started to show any more definite symptoms of the leukaemia, there was no urgent need to get her on chemotherapy.

I did feel quite sorry for them. They'd come in with a healthy dog suffering from a mild case of hair loss and lack of energy and were told that it was probably a minor problem, but were then suddenly confronted with the terrible diagnosis of blood cancer. I suppose cases like this show the benefit of taking routine blood tests. If we hadn't found the leukaemia, it may not have been diagnosed until she was showing fairly advanced symptoms of the disease, when it could have been too late to help her. At least now the correct diagnosis has been made, we can get her on the treatment as soon as any symptoms appear, which should give her the best possible chance of survival.

Sunday 14 December

8.30 p.m. Cheltenham I got home to find that the bloody kittens have brought home another hand puppet! It's Sooty, beautifully made from soft furry cloth and obviously a cherished child's toy. I wish we knew where they were getting them from because there must be a very upset child somewhere wondering why their beloved collection of puppets is gradually disappearing!

Tuesday 16 December

9.15 a.m. Darren has just rung up to ask if I want to go up and do a cruciate op with him this morning as they've got one in. I was planning to do some grassboard testing, but I think learning how to do a cruciate repair would be a better way to spend the day. I told him that I would come straight up.

I assume I won't get paid for coming in, but it's for my own benefit anyway, so it's worth doing. Once I've done this one with Darren's help, I should be able to do them on my own, which is a good skill to have.

1.30 p.m. Halesowen One cruciate repaired! The dog (an elderly spaniel which had ruptured the ligament jumping over a stile) was already anaesthetized and prepped when I arrived, and Darren was waiting to start.

I scrubbed up and put on the sterile gown and gloves which are standard apparel here for all major ops, and placed the drapes around the site where I would make the incision. With Darren's guidance I cut down through the skin and underlying tissue to expose the tendon from which the new ligament graft is taken. The next step is the most critical in the operation – cutting a strip off the edge of the tendon and muscle below of exactly the right size. The strip is taken from the edge of the tendon that attaches the knee cap to the tibia (or shin bone in humans). If the new ligament was cut too short or too thin, then there was no second chance, the operation would have to be abandoned.

With a shaking scalpel, I cut out the strip, leaving it attached at the lower end as this would remain anchored to the tibia when the graft formed the new ligament. Next, I opened up the knee joint and removed the debris of the ruptured ligament and damaged cartilage. It was amazing to see the two split ends of the ligament inside the joint, just how it's described in the textbooks.

After tidying up the inside of the joint, the next phase of the operation was to pass the graft through the joint and suture it to the back of the femur. This is done using a special instrument called a graft passer, which is basically a hook with a hole in it. According to what I'd read and been told about the operation, passing the hook through the joint from the back is the hardest part of the operation, so I was expecting to have to struggle a bit before I got the graft in place. However, I think I must have been very lucky, because on only the second attempt the graft passer slipped through the joint and appeared in the correct place. Once the graft was in place, it was just a matter of firmly stitching it in, checking that the joint was now stable but could still move, and closing up all the various layers which had been cut through on the way in.

The op took just over an hour, which wasn't too bad. I was happy with the end result and Darren seemed to think it had gone pretty well. The proof of success won't come for about a month or so though, by which time the joint should be pretty much back to how it was before the accident.

Now I've done this one with a little help (Darren held a few things out of the way and generally guided me through what to cut and what not to cut) I should be able to tackle one on my own, although it'll still be pretty nerve-racking. It's not the kind of op I'd want to make a mess of because the consequences (permanent lameness) could be pretty serious.

If Pan ruptured his cruciate I don't think I'd do the op because I'd be too upset if I made a mess of it. I suppose I shouldn't be willing to operate on other people's pets if I'm not confident enough to do it on my own, but it is slightly different, operating on your own animal. I'd get Emma to do it!

I checked with Darren about Zoe's progress, and he said they'd decided to leave her and not do anything with the fractured bones because she's looking fine.

4.20 p.m. Got home to find an owl, Sweep and a pair of child's socks on the floor. Bloody kittens!

7.20 p.m. Dad's just rung up to discuss what we're doing for Christmas. I said that he should come down here because we'd like to spend our first Christmas living together in our house, so it looks like he'll come down on Christmas Eve and stay for a few days, which will be excellent.

I haven't seen Dad for ages, not since I was in Bideford, so it's about time we met up again. I also rang Sam, my brother, to see if he and Nicola could come as well, and he said that as long as his band haven't got any gigs lined up, they should be able to. I haven't seen them for even longer, so it should be a brilliant Christmas if they all make it.

Emma's just got in from evening surgery and I've made

a dubious-looking Spanish omelette for dinner. She doesn't look overly impressed!

11.45 p.m. Binned the omelette and went to the pub for steak and chips and a few pints instead! Much better idea than stodgy omelette and boring TV.

Thursday 18 December

Hard day at Halesowen. Lots of consulting.

Home to find unidentifiable but possibly crocodile hand puppet being chewed on the floor by guilty looking Pan!

I went for a look around the houses which back on to the car park behind our bungalow, but no sign of any notes offering rewards for the safe return of Sooty, Sweep and animal friends. I asked one of our neighbours (not entirely on good terms because of an unfortunate dog poo incident a few weeks ago) if he's missing any hand puppets, but no joy. I might have to fit a small video camera to Nigel's head and record where he goes on his stealing missions. If this carries on much longer we'll be able to open a puppet emporium!

Friday 19 December

Exciting grassboard development!!

I got a phone call from work saying that someone from a plastics company was trying to get in contact with me, and could I ring them back. The company is called West Midlands Mouldings, and according to Mr Jones, who I spoke to, they make all sorts of plastic and fibreglass things ranging from trains to sinks. Mr Jones said he'd heard me talking about the grassboard on the radio last week and thought that they might be able to help me develop it.

I'm going up to see them on Monday. It sounds too good to be true – I knew something would come of that interview!

It'll be fantastic if they can make a proper, moulded board because although it works well at the moment, I don't think it looks quite professional enough to market.

No more puppets today, thank God! I think the supply might be running out. Either that, or the owners have got wise to what's going on and have erected some defences to keep out unwanted intruders. Nigel and Brian contented themselves with batting all our pens under the sofa and then mewing continually when they couldn't get them out again. Although they do have their cute, cuddly moments, they are almost more trouble than they're worth. It would be very easy to make them disappear, I could just tell Emma that they must have been run over, or captured in enemy puppet territory and she'd never know the dark truth.

Only joking! They might be nothing but trouble, but I wouldn't go so far as to put them to sleep. Permanently sedate them maybe!

Saturday 20 December

8.35 a.m. Halesowen Start of another two days of hard labour. The BBC are supposed to be here, but no sign of them yet.

8.55 a.m. Amanda, Emma and the crew arrived after apparently being stuck outside the Michael Wood services for three-quarters of an hour. I reckon it was a late-night BBC piss-up last night myself!

12.30 a.m. No decent BBC stories. There was one case that really got me angry though. It was a woman called Mrs Hartbury-Smith, who breeds Dobermanns. She brought in a six-week-old puppy because it had an infected tail stump where it'd been docked.

'Oh, they all get a bit of it, but this one just won't clear up, and I've got some interested people coming to look at him next week,' she said, obviously far more concerned with the outcome of the sale than with the puppy's welfare. 'I'll have some Synulox for him, that usually clears it up in a couple of days.'

I was getting more and more annoyed by this stage. Firstly, this stuck-up, know-it-all woman brings in a puppy which has got a horrible infected tail stump because she had it docked just to make it suitable for showing, and then she has the nerve to tell me what to treat it with.

'That's very nasty,' I said in as unfriendly a tone as I could manage while I examined the puppy. The poor little thing had a large discharging abscess where the base of his tail should have been, and was obviously in a lot of pain and discomfort. All because some bloody organization has decided that Dobermanns look nice without tails.

'It's going to need at least a week of antibiotics, and if that doesn't clear it up, we may have to drain it surgically. It really shouldn't have been allowed to get into this state.'

'Well, in a perfect world, I suppose not, but when you've got three pedigree litters on the go at once things can get missed, you know?' Her tone of voice implied that I really should have more understanding about the difficulties of rearing not just any old mongrels but show-winning pedigree dogs. It was obvious things like this probably happen to her animals all the time and she thinks it's quite acceptable. I mean, what else could she do? The dogs must be docked if they're going to win shows and make her lots of money, so they have to put up with the suffering.

I considered saying exactly what I thought about tail docking (and dog breeding in general), but it was clear she wouldn't listen to me – I mean I'm just her vet, there to supply her with antibiotics and do as she demands. If I'd started to tell her what I really thought about the way she looked after her animals, she would have ended up complaining to Darren or Paul, and possibly going somewhere else. She certainly wouldn't have listened to what I said and changed what she did.

I ended up sending her away with the most expensive

antibiotic we've got. Maybe if compassion and veterinary advice won't change what she does, big vet bills might.

It really does piss me off the way people exploit pets for their own gain. The Mrs Hartbury-Smiths of this world mutilate new-born puppies for the sole reason that they want them to win glory and money in the show ring. Some breeders breed their animals in such a way that they become so deformed they can hardly breath or walk, and are so inbred they're frequently ill and suffer from all sorts of inherited diseases. Bulldogs for example, that symbol of British fighting spirit, are born with such a deformed head they spend their entire life fighting for breath, not for their country. Toy breeds like Pekes and pugs are so badly designed by man that they live in constant pain from sore eyes, bad teeth and bad skin.

What really annoys me is the way in which some breeders will try to justify their animals' grotesque appearance by saying things like, 'Oh, his jaw is supposed to jut out like that. It's because boxers were bred to attack bulls and they needed to have a jaw like that to be able to bite their hide.' Even if this very unlikely fact were true, it's no justification for people to keep on breeding animals that have such unnatural deformities.

Tail docking is one of the worst instances of this kind of thinking. Most breeders of dogs like spaniels or terriers will claim they must be docked so that the tail doesn't get damaged when the dog goes chasing animals through brambles. This is rubbish. For a start, 99 per cent of these dogs will spend most of their time at home or in the show ring, not scrabbling through the undergrowth. Working dogs with tails which do work in thick bushes very, very rarely get any problems from damaging their tails, certainly not enough to justify cutting them off.

Some breeders, such as Mrs Hartbury-Smith, wouldn't even pretend they were docking the dogs for their own protection, they just claim they would look silly if they were left with a tail. What a load of crap! They would only look silly because people are used to seeing them without tails. If they were allowed to have tails, any docked animals would very quickly be the ones which looked out of place.

I always feel so sorry for animals with docked tails because not only have they been through an extremely painful and potentially risky 'operation', but also they have to live their life without being able to communicate properly with other dogs, as the tail is one of the most important means of communication between dogs.

One of the best things that the Royal College has done in the last few years is to ban vets from docking animals' tails, unless for medical reasons. However, even with this ban in place, millions of tails are still being docked across the country, mainly by older vets who refuse to change their ways and are prepared to flout the ban, or by amateurs such as breeders. So, in a way, by banning vets from docking tails, the Royal College could have increased the numbers of puppies suffering as a result of bad docking. I still think they were right to place the ban though – the majority of the dog-loving public are not going to accept such barbaric behaviour from their vets. We are here to help animals and heal them, not to hack bits off them because some people think it looks good.

There goes my lunch-time again. I really must stop getting so carried away when I'm writing my diary at work. I find it very hard to stop myself once I get started. People like Mrs Hartbury-Smith get me so wound up I just have to get it out of my system somehow, and this is the only way that I can think of which doesn't involve actual bodily harm or me being fired!

6.30 p.m. Not a bad afternoon. A few really nice clients, which was just what I needed after this morning.

One interesting case, which the BBC filmed, was a snake with an abscess. It was brought in by a nice woman of fortyish and her teenage son. The snake was in a brown cardboard box, so I was unsure what to expect when I opened it up. This was the first snake I've ever had to treat and that, combined with my inherent fear of all things cold and slimy, made me more than a little apprehensive as I lifted the lid.

Inside was a greeny-brown snake about a metre in length and an inch in diameter.

'Hello, Gizmo,' said the son, reaching in to pick up the snake.

'Er, what type of snake is he?' I asked, eyeing the evil-looking mouth for signs of venomous fangs.

'He's a Californian King,' announced the son proudly, as Gizmo slithered through his hands.

Unfortunately, my knowledge of snakes is second only to my knowledge of spiders in its weakness, so the title Californian King snake did nothing to dissolve my fear of being bitten and dying in agony from lethal venom.

I decided to assume that, as the mother was looking happily at her son as he handled the snake, probably wasn't poisonous. As a precaution I thought it best if the snake stayed in his hands while I examined it from a safe distance.

'He's got a lump on his head,' explained the boy when I asked what the problem was. 'I noticed it yesterday, didn't I, Mum?'

'Yes, and it seems to have grown overnight. He doesn't want to eat now does he, Rob?'

'No. I offered him a mouse this morning and he didn't want to know – usually he eats them straight away.'

I peered at Gizmo's tiny wedge-shaped head and could immediately see the lump in question. Even with my poor knowledge of the anatomy of snakes' heads I realized that the swelling above the right eye was abnormal. Unfortunately, although I could tell it was abnormal, I had no idea what it could be. I decided to abandon professional pride and go and look in the *Manual of Exotic Pets*. This was one case I couldn't bluff my way through.

I excused myself, saying I was just going to have a quick look through a textbook for some clues as to Gizmo's problem, and went through into the corridor where the emergency textbooks are kept (carefully positioned so that all the vets can get to them in times of crisis). To my surprise, when I looked under snakes, one of the few clinical conditions listed was the sub-specular abscess, which, according to the book, presents as a swelling above the eye. I quickly read through the information on the condition and its treatment, and went back to the consulting room to announce my diagnosis.

'It looks as though the swelling is probably an abscess,' I said, trying to look as if I had suspected that all along. 'What we need to do is give him an anaesthetic and lance it. We'll also send away a sample from the fluid in the abscess to the lab to find out which antibiotic will be best to treat it with.'

The boy looked worried, and asked if Gizmo was going to be OK.

'I hope so,' I replied. 'But there is a small risk with all anaesthetics. He's got to have the operation, though, because it won't get better otherwise.'

I didn't tell him that this would be my first snake anaesthetic.

I'm going to read up on snake anaesthetics this evening!

Sunday 21 December

1.15 p.m. Morning surgery done, time for Gizmo's op. The BBC are over the moon about this story because it should make pretty interesting viewing if things go to plan – and extremely interesting viewing if they don't!

1.20 p.m. Just given him an anaesthetic injection in the muscle. It's a drug usually used in cats, but the book assures me that it's OK in snakes.

1.30 p.m. Still very much awake.

1.45 p.m. Thought he was dozing off, but when I touched him, he slithered away in a very conscious manner. I think the injection should have had a bit more effect by now.

1.55 p.m. Just rung up an exotic animal vet in Stafford for advice (a vet who treats exotic animals, that is, not an exotic vet). He said that Saffan, the drug I used, was very variable and often didn't work at all. He suggested I should give a different anaesthetic, in the vein this time instead of the muscle. I admitted to him that I wasn't overly practised in the art of intravenous injections in snakes, so he explained where the best vein is to be found and the technique of injecting into it. It's very useful being able to talk to specialist vets at times like this, and most vets are more than happy to give out advice to beleaguered colleagues in times of need.

1.57 p.m. Right, injection ready, with the smallest needle I could find. How hard can it be to find a snake's tail vein?

2.10 p.m. Bloody hard!

2.16 p.m. Finally got at least some of the injection into the vein, after trying for twenty minutes. Having the cameras peering over my shoulder the whole time didn't help, nor did the fact that although Gizmo isn't very big, he can certainly struggle like the biggest python.

In the end it took three nurses to hold him still, and even with him semi-immobilized, finding the vein was far from straightforward. According to the specialist, the vein should have been lying just under the scales of the tail, but it took lots of blind stabs with the needle before I hit any blood. Then, even when I knew roughly where the vein was, it took several more attempts before I was happy that the needle was in the vein. When I injected the drug, a white liquid used in humans as well as animals, some went into the vein, but then he moved and the rest squirted over his scales.

I don't know if I've got enough in or not, just have to wait and see if he goes to sleep.

2.24 p.m. Hooray! He's finally showing some signs of dozing off. I managed to touch him without him slithering away, but he's still not fully asleep because as I touched his tail he eyed me with his little yellow eyes as if to say, 'Any closer and there'll be trouble!' I may have read that Californian King snakes are totally harmless, but I'm still not taking any chances with him!

2.35 p.m. All done. He got more and more sleepy until he was quiet enough for me to be able to lance the swelling with a tiny needle. I drew off about 0.5 ml of cloudy fluid, which I put into a sterile tube so it could be sent off to the lab for analysis, and then flushed out the abscess with sterile water and dilute antibiotics. A success, after a worrying start!

2.37 p.m. Oh, no! He's just gone limp and stopped breathing – I think he might be dead!

3.00 p.m. Jesus, what a stressful few minutes!

Just as I was beginning to panic, Caroline, one of the nurses who had been helping to hold him, said she could see a heartbeat. I looked where she was pointing, and to my immense relief I could see a small area on the side of Gizmo's body wall pulsing slowly. A faint heartbeat wasn't enough though, unless he was breathing, the heart would stop pretty quickly.

I decided in a flash of inspiration what I needed to do was to get a tube into his windpipe somehow so we could breathe for him until he recovered consciousness enough to take over himself. I frantically searched through the drawers until I found a small intravenous catheter. I pulled off the sterile wrapping and took the metal stilette out, leaving just the plastic tube with its attached hub. I grabbed Gizmo's head and looked inside his mouth. I had no idea about the anatomy of a snake's mouth, but it was quite obvious when

I looked that the small opening on the floor of the mouth must be the opening to the snake equivalent of the windpipe. The small plastic catheter slid straight into the opening, and I immediately brought my mouth down on to the hub and blew gently through the tube. As I blew, I could see Gizmo's flank gently rise and fall – the tube must be in the right place I thought with relief.

After a few breaths I stood back to see if he was going to breathe alone and to everyone's surprise, after about a minute, his flanks rose and fell as he took a tiny breath through the catheter.

He's now on a blanket with a hot-water bottle, with Caroline giving him breaths of oxygen using the smallest anaesthetic circuit connected up to the catheter.

I think what must have happened is that the first anaesthetic kicked in after I gave him the intravenous one and the two combined have overdosed him. Now it's just going to be a matter of keeping him alive until he can get the drugs out of his system.

The BBC have recorded the whole episode. Amanda's just admitted that she's been torn between feeling bad for the snake and me, and feeling excited as the story unfolded. If he makes it through, it's going to be an amazing story – vet giving snake the kiss of life!

4.45 p.m. Gizmo still unconscious and being ventilated by Caroline. I'm still very worried – what will I tell Rob if he dies?

6.00 p.m. Still no movement. His heart rate has increased a bit, which is a good sign, but he's still only breathing on his own every few minutes.

6.24 p.m. He moved! Caroline called me through from doing surgery and said that she'd seen his jaw twitch and his tail move a tiny bit. He didn't move while I was watching so I hope she was right and didn't imagine it.

6.36 p.m. Definite signs of life. His jaw moved a couple of times and his tail moved across the blanket about two inches (although that could have been me moving the blanket).

7.01 p.m. He's alive and waking up! He's breathing on his own so Caroline has taken the tube out, and he's slowly moving. I've never been so happy to see a snake slither!

7.45 p.m. I'm off home at last. I was supposed to finish at 6.00, but I didn't want to leave until I was happy that Gizmo was going to be OK. He's pretty much awake now, although still very slow and groggy. I can't believe what a disaster his anaesthetic has been. The whole procedure should have taken about twenty minutes, but instead the whole practice has been in a state of red alert for over six hours!

One thing is very certain – I am not going to become a snake expert!

9.00 p.m. Home to find two pairs of children's socks and a squirrel puppet on the floor. Something has got to be done about our bloody kittens!

10.15 p.m. Told Emma the snake saga. She thought it was most amusing. I suppose it might seem funny to me in a few weeks, but right now I'm just so relieved that he survived.

Monday 22 December

7.30 p.m. Last day at Halesowen before Christmas. Quite busy, but no BBC so not too stressful. Gizmo was alive and back to full slither thankfully. I didn't tell his owners about the little trouble we had with the anaesthetic, I didn't think it was worth getting them upset. He survived with no ill effects after all, although I know it could have been very different. I thanked Caroline for spending all yesterday afternoon nursing Gizmo through my messed-up anaesthetic – I think it was a combination of luck and her efforts which got him through it.

During the couple of hours which I had off between surgeries today, I went over to West Midlands Mouldings to meet Mr Jones and see what they could do with the grass-board. The factory is in a big old industrial building in the middle of a rundown industrial estate next to a railway line, only a few miles from the practice. I met Mr Jones, who turned out to be an elderly man dressed in a faded brown suit. The whole place gave off an air of age and looked to be in need of updating.

However, he seemed very interested in the board, and explained that his company specializes in making fibreglass mouldings. He seems to think that they should be able to make a moulded one-piece board with the right flexibility and strength characteristics using either fibreglass and resin, or flexible epoxy resins, which is what the deck is made out of at the moment.

He said they would look into the best method of making the board early in the new year, and then if it looked feasible, they should be able to get me a prototype within a few months. I explained that I really want to get the board developed and ready to sell by next spring, because otherwise the rival MBS board will have too much of a head start, even if it is as inferior as I think.

It's an exciting development though. I really hope it works out because I've put so much effort into getting the board this far, it'd be awful if it doesn't make it to production.

Dad has just rung to say that he and Sam and Nicola are all definitely coming for Christmas, which is going to be excellent. It'll also give me a good chance to try and persuade Dad to invest in the grassboard project!

I'd better go shopping for presents, I haven't bought any yet (as usual for me). I haven't got a clue what to get Emma. I think I should get her something really romantic and different because we've not been seeing that much of each other recently, what with me working in Birmingham, and I feel we need to rekindle some of the old passion in the relationship.

Tuesday 23 December

Went shopping in Cheltenham today, this is what I bought:

> Emma – Two CDs (no romantic presents to be had
> for love nor money in Cheltenham, need
> inspiration and fast)
> Dad – Car fire extinguisher (as requested, not
> exciting but what he wants)
> Sam – Obscure vinyl LP
> Nicola – Delegated to Emma – (thought about an
> antique collection of children's hand puppets
> but decided against it)
> Mum – T-shirt, sent off to France today, should
> arrive mid-January

Emma's gone into a cleaning frenzy this evening. I tried to tell her that my family are more than used to living in squalid conditions, but she's come over all houseproud, and wants the place looking spotless for when they arrive tomorrow.

Wednesday 24 December Christmas Eve

I had present inspiration in the bath last night. I've organized Emma a day's rally driving at Brands Hatch, which is right next to her home in Kent. I think she'll love it. She's always going on about wanting to slide her car around and have a go in a proper rally car. The only problem is that it's quite expensive so I won't be able to have a go as well. It's going to be awful watching her getting to drive a 200 bhp Cosworth while I sit on the sidelines. I suppose that's love though!

Dad and Sam and Nicola should be here soon. Emma's cracked open the first bottle of wine, so it looks like being a good night!

9.15 p.m. Hic, things going well. Dad and Sam and Nicola all here OK. On bottle of wine number three I think. Ham still cooking.

10.10 p.m. Ham finally ready, wine nearly gone. Might have to resort to remains of Jake Johnson's whisky from Bideford.

11.20 p.m. Whisky slippin' down nicely. Ham was great.

11.45 a.m. I'm getting married!! Emma's jus' proposed an' I said yes! I was gonna do it soon, but she beat me to it . . . anyway, end result's same – we're gerring married! Dad an' Sam v. happy.

Thursday 25 December Christmas Day

10.30 a.m. Oooh!

11.00 a.m. Oooh! Not feeling the best. Need tea.

11.35 a.m. Up, feeling better with a couple of cups of tea on board.

11.38 a.m. Bloody hell! I've just remembered that I'm engaged!

It's a bit of a shock, but I think I'm very happy. It's been on the cards for ages, but I kept not getting round to asking her, so in the end I think she just got fed up with waiting and asked me instead.

She was convinced I would have changed my mind by this morning, but now I'm getting used to the idea, I'm very happy with it. I can't see myself ever wanting anyone else, which I suppose is the sign that you're ready to get married.

Anyway, I gave her a ring last night so it's official. Admittedly the ring was drunkenly fashioned from tinfoil and Sellotape, but it's the thought that counts. I'll get her a decent one as soon as possible, although personally I can't see what's wrong with the tinfoil one, much cheaper to insure than diamonds!

3.00 p.m. Em very happy with present. She got me some CDs and a superb watch. Wine is open again (Dad's restocked the wine rack), so I might make this my last entry today, otherwise my diary will fill up with even more drunken rubbish!

Friday 26 December Boxing Day

7.00 p.m. It's been an excellent Christmas. We all went up to Cleeve Hill today, and I demonstrated the grassboard, and we walked the mutts (who are both much too fat after three days of drunken titbits from the table). Dad said he'll invest in the grassboard, which is fantastic of him. I just hope it isn't a great disaster which loses loads of money!

Sam and Nicola have just gone back to Cambridge because Sam's band, The Babysitters, are doing a gig in London tomorrow. I've heard them play live a couple of times and they are really good. He gave us a CD which they've just had recorded and it's bloody impressive. I hope they make it big time. They deserve to because Sam's got so much talent at writing songs and he's pretty useful on the guitar as well.

I wrote a song when I was at college called The Curry Song, which went something like, 'It's Wednesday night and I'm going for a curry. It's open till three so there ain't no hurry.' It had three chords and was truly awful! Sam definitely got the musical talent in our family!

Emma, Dad and me are off down the pub to round off a great few days with a couple of little pints.

Wednesday 31 December New Year's Eve

4.30 p.m. Just got back from spending a couple of nights in Devon with Emma. We stayed in a pub in Croyde and had an excellent romantic time, and I got a bit of surfing in, although the water was freezing and my wet suit is full of holes.

Tonight we might go to the pub later on, but we're going to spend most of the evening lying in front of the fire in the living room under the duvet watching some videos. We've both decided, since we got engaged, that we need to spend more time together and enjoy ourselves, so we're going to have a romantic evening doing just that.

11.00 p.m. Off to the pub to see the New Year in. It's been great, just being here together on our own this evening.

1.20 p.m. Emma's asleep, but I'm just going to stay up for a few more minutes. I'm in one of those mellow, chilled-out moods where I don't feel sleepy, and just want to relax and think about life and the last year.

I feel as if I've come a long way in the last twelve months, as a vet, and in other ways. A year ago I was still unsure about what I wanted in my life and was content to drift along with no real direction, but now I feel so much happier and I know what I want in the future. The best thing, by far, has been realizing how much I love Emma and finally convincing myself that marriage is not a one-way ticket to a mortgage and a dull settled existence, but is just a way of saying that we know we are right for each other and we're going to stay together. It won't stop me going surfing, or grassboarding, or any of the other things I want to do, it'll just mean that instead of going through life on my own, I'll be in a partnership.

We decided while we were away that we're going to get married this summer. Neither of us see the point in waiting, now that we've finally made the decision. We're going to have a small registry-office wedding and a massive party at my dad's house. Neither of us are at all religious, and we both hate the idea of a big expensive traditional wedding, so we're going to concentrate on making the reception a party to remember!

I wonder if Ian and Keith will come to the wedding – it'd be great to see them again. Every now and then I get a big surge of sadness when I think of Bideford, and I some-times wish I'd stayed there. It was such a nice place, and Ian and Keith were so good to me. I know deep down that I made the right decision, because Emma and I are so happy now, both in our new jobs and because we're living together.

I wonder what I'll be writing in this diary in a year's time. I hope I'll be looking back on a year when we had the wedding of the century, and the grassboard took off and developed into a multi-million-pound industry! I also hope that Emma's job continues to be as good as it is, and that I finally find a decent part-time job a bit nearer home. I enjoy working in Halesowen, but I don't think I can keep up the long hours and long drive for that much longer.

Anyway, I'm ready for bed. We're off to Emma's home tomorrow to see her parents. She's got the rally driving booked up for Friday!

August

Sunday 9 August

I'm a married man! After eight months of very lax and disorganized preparation, the big day finally arrived yesterday. We'd decided to have a relaxed, very informal wedding, and concentrate on having a fantastic party that all our friends would remember for a long time. So instead of a big church ceremony and a sit-down reception in a big expensive venue, we had a small registry-office wedding followed by a Hawaiian-style party at my dad's house.

The actual wedding itself was held in a small room in Oundle registry office. It was lovely to have both our families there, especially Mum, who came over from France, and Emma's sister Jo, who flew over from Canada. The ceremony only lasted about quarter of an hour, but it was very emotional and special. The BBC filmed in the room, but were quite discreet!

After the ceremony we had our grand entrance. We arrived at the reception by river, on a raft, as my dad's house is on the river and the reception was Hawaiian. We thought it would be much more fitting to arrive by water rather than in the traditional limo, so we borrowed a raft from the local sailing club and decorated it with flowers and reeds. Jim and Jon, our witnesses/best men paddled us down the river from a secret mooring, and we arrived to the theme music of *Hawaii-five-O*. We'd kept the arrival secret so all the guests were pretty surprised when they saw us. It was fantastic, especially as nearly all the hundred or so guests had come in fancy dress, so when we rounded the final corner of the river, we saw a mass of our friends all dressed in wild shirts and garlands of flowers. The sun was shining properly for the first time in the whole summer – it just couldn't have been any better!

The party that followed was amazing. Emma's family and family friends, John and Glenny, had prepared a gourmet buffet, and my mum had brought over a carload of wine from France, so things started on a good note. After the food and wine, we had a few speeches, and then as it started to get dark, my brother's band, The Babysitters, played outside. As the band finished, we had one of the highlights of the evening – a firework display over the river.

The disco started up after the fireworks and the party carried on into the early hours of the morning. Well, quite late hours to be exact – I think me and Emma got to bed around five!

We all feel pretty poor this morning, but it was well worth the hangover. We took a risk having such an unconventional reception, but I think everyone had an excellent time. I know Emma and I did. We'll always remember yesterday as one of the happiest days of our lives; just being there with all our friends, everyone enjoying themselves, was the best feeling in the world.

We've got a week back at work now before we're off on our honeymoon because next Saturday is the British All-terrain Boarding Championships. I managed to persuade Emma that we should delay our holiday by a week so I could enter, and to my surprise she agreed without a struggle. I think she can see that at last the grassboard is looking as if it is going to take off after all the months of disappointments. It's been very frustrating, mainly thanks to West Midlands Mouldings, who have failed miserably in their attempts to make a moulded deck for the board. After waiting and waiting for months and months for any progress they finally produced a board that snapped as soon as any pressure was put on it. 'Not to worry,' they said. 'Just as few minor adjustments to the resin mix and it'll be fine.' Six months later they're still no nearer coming up with a useable board, so I've had to go back to the old idea of a flat deck with metal endplates. This works fine, but doesn't look as good as a moulded deck would do.

Apart from the difficulties with the actual production of

the board, everything else has been going really well. Pete, an old surfing friend, has been riding with me a lot, and we've made several advances in the design of the board. As a result, we've been going down hills and doing tricks that I never thought would be possible on a grassboard, such as 360° spins and board-slides along metal rails. We're both convinced that the sport is going to take off, it's just a matter of how we make the board and whether it can be made into a viable business.

Sunday 16 August

Yesterday was fantastic. NO SNO (as we've called the company) wiped out the opposition and me, Pete and Jim (my best man) came first, second and third in all the events!

It was organized by the UK distributors of the American board, and I think they were pretty annoyed that we came along and completely outclassed them. There was a downhill slalom, a freestyle jumping contest, and the border-cross, which is basically a free-for-all race with a few obstacles in the way.

We made several good contacts and I think a lot of the other competitors and spectators were pretty impressed. Hopefully, once we're finally ready to start selling the boards, people will remember today and buy NO SNO rather than the opposition.

Emma and I are just about to leave for Gatwick on our honeymoon. We're going to the Dominican Republic for two weeks of sun and relaxation. Both of us are desperate just to have some time alone together without all the stress of weddings, grassboards and being vets.

The wedding was fantastic, but what with organizing it, and trying to get the grassboards ready for yesterday, and being busy at work, life has been a little hectic over the last month or so, to say the least. Two weeks away with nothing to do and nothing to worry about is going to be just what the doctor ordered, or should that be 'just what the *vet* ordered'!